Dr N Macmillan

RESPIRATORY DISEASES

MANAGEMENT OF COMMON DISEASES IN FAMILY PRACTICE

Series Editors: J. Fry and M. Lancaster-Smith

RESPIRATORY DISEASES

G. Jariwalla, MB, BCh (Wales), MRCP
Consultant Physician, Bromley and Tunbridge Wells Health Authorities, Kent

Contributions from:
John Fry, OBE, MD, FRCS, FRCGP
General Practitioner, Beckenham, Kent

and

H. Hutchinson, MB, MRCS, DA, FFA, RCS
Consultant Anaesthetist, Tunbridge Wells Health Authority
(chapter on Terminal Illness)

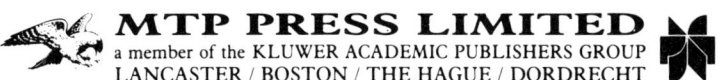

MTP PRESS LIMITED
a member of the KLUWER ACADEMIC PUBLISHERS GROUP
LANCASTER / BOSTON / THE HAGUE / DORDRECHT

Published in the UK and Europe by
MTP Press Limited
Falcon House
Lancaster, England

British Library Cataloguing in Publication Data

Jariwalla, G.
 Respiratory diseases – (Management of common diseases in family practice)
 1. Respiratory organs – Diseases
 I. Title II. Fry, J. III. Hutchinson, H. IV. Series
 616.2   RC731

ISBN 0-85200-757-4

Copyright © 1985 G. Jariwalla

All rights reserved. No part of this publication may be reproduced, stored in a retrieval system, or transmitted in any form or by any means, electronic, mechanical, photocopying, recording or otherwise, without prior permission from the publishers.

Typeset by UPS Blackburn, 76-80 Northgate, Blackburn, Lancashire.
Printed by Butler and Tanner Ltd., Frome and London.

Contents

	Series Editors' Foreword	vii
	Acknowledgements	viii
1.	Background	1
2.	Symptoms and their management	2
3.	Radiological investigations	42
4.	Catarrhal children	53
5.	Chronic bronchitis and emphysema	59
6.	Bronchial asthma	73
7.	Tumours of the lung	100
8.	Management of terminal illness	128
9.	Tuberculosis	148
10.	Sarcoidosis	162
11.	Acute infections of the lungs	168

12.	Chronic infections of the lungs	181
13.	Fibrotic lung disorders	195
14.	Emergencies	206
	Multiple Choice Questions	212
	Index	217

Series Editors' Foreword

Effective management logically follows accurate diagnosis. Such logic often is difficult to apply in practice. Absolute diagnostic accuracy may not be possible, particularly in the field of primary care, when management has to be on analysis of symptoms and on knowledge of the individual patient and family.

This series follows that on *Problems in Practice* which was concerned more with diagnosis in the widest sense and this series deals more definitively with general care and specific treatment of symptoms and diseases.

Good management must include knowledge of the nature, course and outcome of the conditions, as well as prominent clinical features and assessment and investigations, but the emphasis is on what to do best for the patient.

Family medical practitioners have particular difficulties and advantages in their work. Because they often work in professional isolation in the community and deal with relatively small numbers of near-normal patients their experience with the more serious and more rare conditions is restricted. They find it difficult to remain up-to-date with medical advances and even more difficult to decide on the suitability and application of new and relatively untried methods compared with those that are 'old' and well proven.

Their advantages are that because of long-term continuous care for their patients they have come to know them and their families well and are able to become familiar with the more common and less serious diseases of their communities.

This series aims to correct these disadvantages by providing practical information and advice on the less common, potentially serious conditions, but at the same time to take note of the special features of general medical practice.

To achieve these objectives, the *titles* are intentionally those of accepted body systems and population groups.

The *co-authors* are a specialist and a family practitioner so that each can supplement and complement the other.

The *experience bases* are those of the district general hospital and family practice. It is here that the day-to-day problems arise.

The *advice and presentation* are practical and have come from many years of conjoint experience of family and hospital practice.

The *series* is intended for family practitioners – the young and the less than young. All should benefit and profit from comparing the views of the authors with their own. Many will coincide, some will be accepted as new, useful and worthy of application and others may not be acceptable, but nevertheless will stimulate thought and enquiry.

Since medical care in the community and in hospitals involves teamwork, this series also should be of relevance to nurses and others involved in personal and family care.

JOHN FRY
M. LANCASTER-SMITH

Acknowledgements

My sincere appreciation of my wife Lynne's patience and many thanks to Mrs. Mary Evans and Melanie Ray for typing the manuscript.

1

Background

☐☐☐☐☐☐☐☐☐☐☐

BACKGROUND

Respiratory diseases constitute a very significant proportion of ailments presenting in general practice.

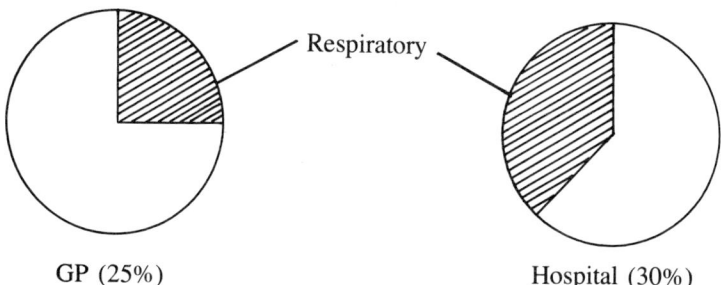

GP (25%)　　　　　　　　Hospital (30%)

Prevalence of respiratory disorders

Approximately one quarter of the work is with some aspect of respiratory diseases[1]. One third of acute medical admissions to a district general hospital are 'respiratory'.

Upper respiratory tract infections are very common in childhood. These may result in the so-called 'wheezy child' – a syndrome difficult to distinguish from bronchial asthma.

RESPIRATORY DISEASES

Chronic bronchitis and emphysema may appear as early as 30 years of age and their incidence is rising amongst females. Young children living in families where members smoke have a higher chance ultimately of developing chronic bronchitis and emphysema. Many bronchitics develop irreversible damage with disability and embarrassment that lead eventually to respiratory failure and cor pulmonale (right heart failure secondary to chronic pulmonary conditions). A patient with chronic bronchitis and emphysema becomes a regular attender at a general practitioner's surgery.

The term *chronic obstructive airways diseases (COAD)* is still used for any respiratory conditions characterized by obstruction and coughing and includes *chronic bronchitis and emphysema* (mainly irreversible), *bronchial asthma* (potentially reversible) and *bronchiectasis* (with partially reversible airways obstruction). Asthma and bronchiectasis are more easily controlled and self-managed by patients.

Chronic obstructive airways disorders (COAD)

Type	Chest X-ray	Features
• *Chronic bronchitis and emphysema* (COMMONEST)	Hyperinflation	• Smoking patient • Male > female

• *Asthma*	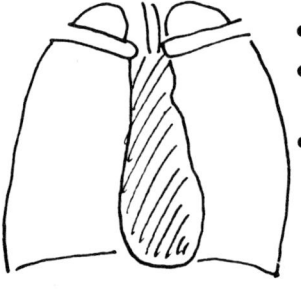
	Hyperinflation
		• Usually non-smoker
		• ? allergy
		  ? Inheritance
		• Male > female (childhood)
		  Female > males (adults)

BACKGROUND

• *Bronchiectasis*

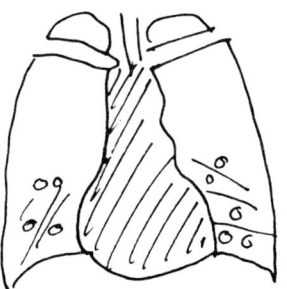

• Previous history of 'chest' trouble
• Males = females
• May be a smoker

Hyperinflation
with increased background shadows

Asthma was known to ancient Greeks as a 'panting' and 'suffocating' disorder. Thomas Willis (1621–75) was among the first to describe bronchiolar constriction, mucosal oedema and sputum plugging. Salter (1964) pioneered the concept of bronchial hypersensitivity. Asthma occurs in up to 5% of the population[2]. Wheezing in children is even more common. These children may belong to a 'smoking' family or be prone to frequent 'viral' upper respiratory disorders. Allergic manifestations and positive family history of asthma, hay fever, eczema would make the diagnosis of extrinsic asthma likely. Management of wheezy bronchitis and asthma in childhood should remain the same (see Chapter 6, Bronchial Asthma).

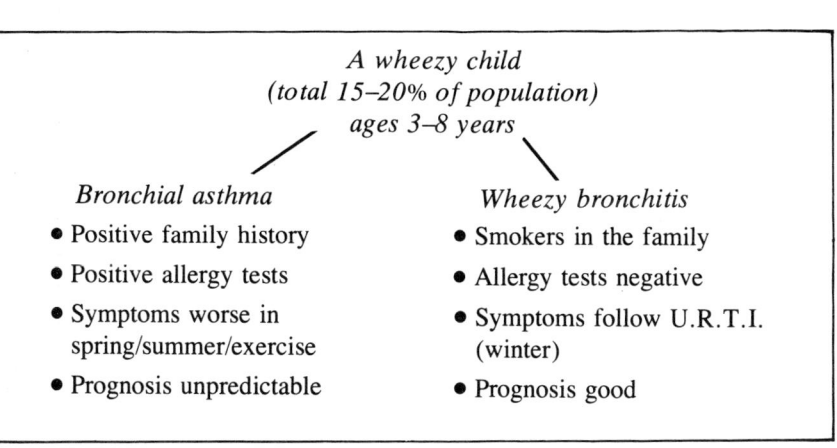

Patient/parent education and explanation is especially important in asthma. A busy general practitioner should recall these patients to a special clinic when he can give 'time'. Detailed explanation must be given on:

- *Aetiology*, prevention
- *Management*: use of inhaler devices and nebulizers
- *Self-recording of PEFR* and charting any variations during the day (Mini-Wright's peak flow meter recommended for 'unstable' asthmatics)
- *When to summon urgent help*

  i.e. $\begin{cases} \text{rapid fall in PEFR} \\ \text{tachypnoea, tachycardia} \\ \text{\& failure to respond to existing therapy} \end{cases}$

- *Possible prognosis*
  (no restrictions in activities in most)

Failure to diagnose, or the misdiagnosis of asthma denies the adult patient/child a means of control of what is a reversible disease. A child will miss schooling and take endless courses of antibiotics. An adult will restrict activities and change his way of life – eventually emphysema may result. Respiratory failure and cor pulmonale are rare in asthma but relatively common in chronic bronchitis and emphysema. The 'misdiagnosed' cases will in time develop these complications as the use of effective bronchodilators (especially steroids) may be limited if asthma is *not* suspected.

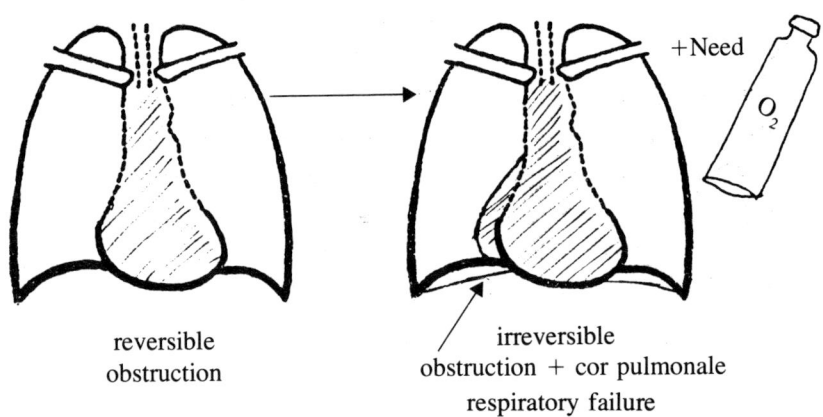

Misdiagnosis of asthma

The reluctance to diagnose asthma – still prevalent – stems from the fear of social stigma and belief that this disease carries a bad prognosis. It is regarded as a disabling disease – however, the patient/relatives should be told of good prognosis in the majority with effective modern therapy. Approximately 1500 deaths are annually attributable to 'asthma' – many preventable.

Occupational lung disorders are increasingly recognized. Some have serious physical and social consequences (e.g. asbestosis = mesothelioma); others are 'nuisance' and may necessitate a change of job! Majority cause lung fibrosis. Some are fatal. Advice should prevent fibrotic and malignant complications in workers involved with mining (including quarry work), asbestos, fibreglass, farming and in a host of common reagents recognized as doing harm to the lungs.

- Coal workers' pneumoconiosis
  (compensatable according to the degree of involvement)
- Asbestosis
  (regular assessment of 'at risk' people may prevent further damage)
- Allergic alveolitis
  (farmers, bakers, housewives (soap powder), veterinary surgeons)

Tuberculosis very rarely presents in the 'old' classical manner of a *wasted, coughing* patient with *haemoptysis* and *night sweats* (*see* Chapter 9, Tuberculosis).

Possible reasons for the decline in TB

- Improved living methods
- BCG (1958)
- Vigilance
- Contact tracing
- ? Routine chest X-rays

70 000 cases in 1920
(England & Wales)
15 000 cases in 1983

There is much discussion on the need to continue BCG (Bacille Calmette–Guérin) vaccination, contact tracing and routine chest X-rays. What effects these measures and possible changes in living standards ± alcohol consumption will have on our future trends cannot be accurately predicted. A general practitioner may see one new case of pulmonary tuberculosis once every 3 years but in areas where there is greater concentration of alcoholics, immigrants and the 'socially deprived' the incidence is greater. A consultant with interest in respiratory diseases may be referred up to 30 new cases per year (average 15–20). Not all patients with tuberculosis are treated by the chest physicians. Extrapulmonary tuberculosis is invariably treated by those who diagnose it, and this often leads to confusion in 'contact tracing'. There is often delay in notification; correct procedure is not followed and in many cases the patients are *not* notified. Delay in undertaking tracing of contacts is somewhat risky and causes a great deal of stress to relatives. The general practitioner should ensure that the practice patients have been notified and contact tracing is in progress. Physicians involved in caring for the chronic ill (especially the geriatric/psychiatric) must be on the lookout for new cases of miliary and postprimary disease.

TB (prevalence)
- GP sees
  1 every 3 years
- Consultant (chest) sees
  20–30 per year

TB (at risk)
- Immigrants
  (Asian, males)
- Alcoholics
- Immunosuppressed

Bronchial carcinoma remains an increasingly difficult problem. In spite of a great deal of health education to persuade the public to give up smoking, there are few signs that the total tobacco consumption has decreased. Over the next 10 years, lung cancer will kill approximately 300 000 patients in the UK. A general practitioner sees only one to two new cases per year and this may give a false impression of infrequence. But there are 30 000 general practitioners in the NHS and the mortality of lung cancer is very high.

Lung cancer
Mortality: 10 years[3]
(UK)
300 000 ✝
(equivalent population London Borough of Bromley)

Lung cancer
GP: 1–2 per year
Consultants
(hospital): 100 per year

Lung cancer
(at risk)
A middle-aged smoking male

Immunological disorders including sarcoidosis are light relief compared with chronic lung diseases, but 1–2% of patients with sarcoidosis and hilar lymphadenopathy may proceed to progressive lung parenchymal involvement. Rheumatoid arthritis, systemic lupus erythematosus (SLE) and polyarteritis nodosa (PAN) may involve the lungs, and prognosis in a particular patient will depend on the extent and progress of lung disease.

BACKGROUND

Immunological lung disorders (common)

Type	*Features*
• Sarcoidosis	
• Rheumatoid arthritis	
• Ankylosing spondylitis	
• SLE/scleroderma	
• Polyarteritis nodosa	

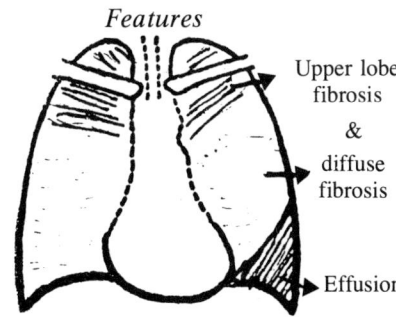

Upper lobe fibrosis & diffuse fibrosis

Effusion

Influenza can produce a devastating effect on a 'weak chest'. Postinfluenzal pneumonia or lower respiratory tract infection may lead to hospital admission. Influenzal vaccination and its ability to prevent influenza is not yet well defined.

There is no doubt that the role of the *'Chest Clinic'* and the attending physician has changed over the past 30 years with emphasis changing from management of tuberculosis to bronchial asthma, carcinoma of the lung and occupational disorders and advice on crippling conditions like chronic bronchitis and emphysema. Although a general practitioner can manage the majority of cases of bronchial asthma and other obstructive airway disorders, some require collaborative care with a specialist. Prevention of smoking and particularly health education at school to prevent children taking up the habit will drastically reduce the incidence of chronic bronchitis, emphysema and lung cancer. Improvement of living standards and prevention of alcoholism will reduce tuberculosis to a minimum. The diligent use of available broncholilators and steroid therapy in conjunction with likely advances in the treatment of asthma will improve their outlook. It is likely that the epidemiology of respiratory disorders in the year 2000 will have a different message to relate.

Future respiratory medicine
- ? Less bronchitis, TB, cancer
- ? Cure for asthma
- ? Prevention of influenza/less pneumonia
- ? Increase occupational disorders

Respiratory disorders can be divided basically into treatable and preventable conditions. Later emphasis is put on management of these conditions.

> *Chronic but ? controllable disorders*
>
> - Asthma
> - Sarcoidosis
> - Collagen disorders
> - Tuberculosis

> *Chronic but potentially preventable*
>
> - Chronic bronchitis and emphysema
> - Occupational disorders
> - Bronchial carcinoma
> - Postinfluenzal infections

References

1. *Studies on Medical and Population Subjects No. 14.* (1958). Morbidity statistics from general practice. Vol. 1. (London: HMSO)
2. Clarke, T. J. H. and Godfrey, S. (eds) (1983). *Epidemiology in Asthma.* (London: Chapman & Hall)
3. Office of Population Censuses and Surveys (1982) (London: HMSO)

2

Symptoms and their management

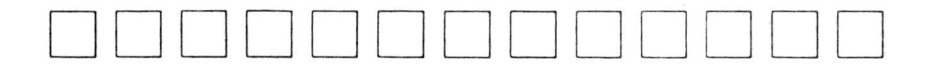

☐ ☐ ☐ ☐ ☐ ☐ ☐ ☐ ☐ ☐ ☐

COUGH

This can be distressing for the patient and socially unacceptable. A coughing child 'disrupts the class'; a bank clerk 'upsets' the customers; in a canteen attendant it is 'unhygienic'; coughing at night keeps the other partner awake. It is the most frequent of the respiratory symptoms leading the patient to seek help.

Significance

> *Coughing children*
> - Common 3–8 years
> - Winter months
> - No cause in many
> - Exclude asthma

- Many children cough during winter. In many no cause will be found.
- A child with cough and persistent wheeze may be asthmatic.
- Over 20% of children have acute wheezy attacks.
- Expectoration of very little or 'glue'-like sputum should make one suspect asthma.
- Detailed history necessary.

RESPIRATORY DISEASES

'Viral' disorders
- Commonest cause of cough
- Constitutional symptoms present

- Viral upper respiratory disorders (colds and influenza) are the commonest cause.
- There will be nasal discharge, sore throat, and viraemia – causing muscle aches, sweating and general malaise.
- Antibiotics only needed in those with evidence of lower respiratory infection with purulent sputum. Beware in glandular fever!

Middle-aged smoker

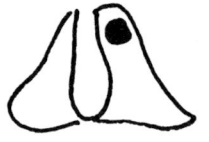

- A middle-aged smoking individual with persistent cough may have lung cancer.
- Chest X-ray necessary. A normal film does not exclude cancer. Either repeat or refer for assessment.

Early chronic bronchitis

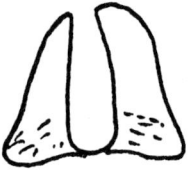

- Early morning cough and sputum – accepted as 'smoker's cough' – may suggest chronic bronchitis, emphysema or bronchiectasis.
- In bronchiectasis – patient will produce large quantities of sputum (often purulent and with haemoptysis.) *NB.* Fibrocytic disease in children.

Nervous 'cough'

!

Diagnosis after exclusion of organic disease

- Cough may be associated with anxiety and 'nerves' – but must not be dismissed as such unless organic conditions have been excluded.
- Patients amazed at the quantity of sputum produced at coughing and questions like 'where is it coming from?' are asked.

Excess sputum
- Chronic airways obstruction
- Physical – foreign body
- Chemical: inhalation
- Infective: pneumonic
- Irritative

- A normal adult produces about 120 ml of mucus per day in the respiratory tract.
- A child with cough and excess sputum: exclude foreign body.

Complications
- Incontinence
- 'Fits'
- Syncope
- Rib fractures

- Persistent cough at night may cause urinary incontinence in very young and old. The cough syncope results from severe bout of coughing leading to raised intracranial pressure interfering with return of blood to the heart. Epileptic convulsions may occur.

COUGH
{
Production of sputum (stimulus of mucus membranes)
- Acute bronchitis
- Bronchiectasis
- Pneumonia
- Bronchial carcinoma

Non-productive (irritation)
- Bronchial asthma
- Viral infections inc. croup
- Allergic and fibrosing alveolitis
- Foreign body, e.g. peanut, dental filling
- Hodgkin's, carcinoid, aneurysm
}

RESPIRATORY DISEASES

Who to investigate

- Persistent
- Haemoptysis
- Smoker
- Chest pain

- A child or adult with persistent cough lasting 3-4 weeks.
- Presence of haemoptysis. It is not always a sinister feature: bronchial carcinoid, pulmonary embolism in a young adult.
- A smoker.
- When accompanied by chest pain, weight loss, night sweats: TB and 'septic' lung conditions.

Evaluation

History
- FAMILY
- HABITS
- OCCUPATION

- Detailed history should include family members with allergic disorders, e.g. hay fever, eczema, asthma.
- Occupational involvement with dust, animals and birds.
- Smoking/alcoholism.
- Inhalation of irritants.

Physical signs

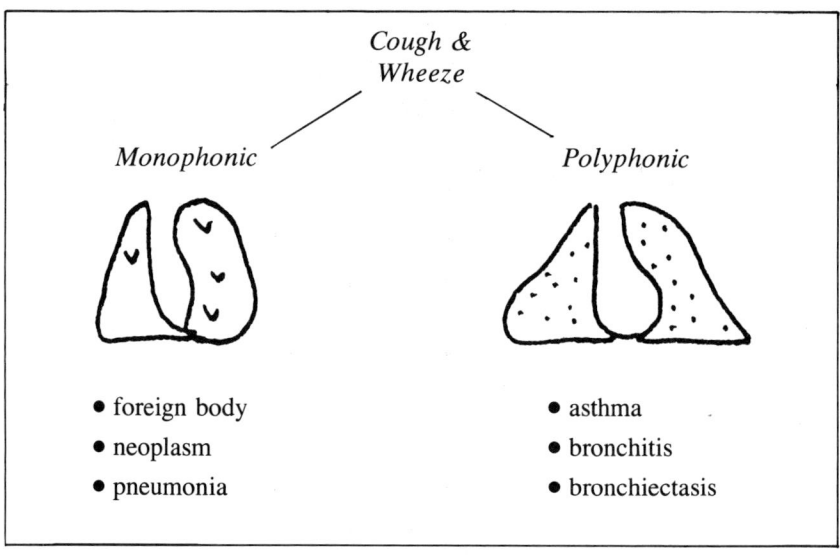

Cough & Wheeze

Monophonic
- foreign body
- neoplasm
- pneumonia

Polyphonic
- asthma
- bronchitis
- bronchiectasis

Cough & Crackles

Generalized (basal)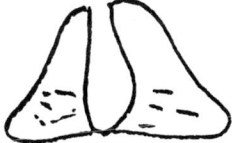

- fibrosis
- viral pneumonia
- heart failure

Localized (apical)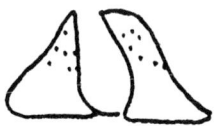

- tuberculosis
- pneumonia (bacterial)
- pulmonary infarction

Tests

Sputum examination
- Asthma stigmata
- Tuberculosis bacilli
- Malignant cells
- Culture (bacterial)

- Microscopic/macroscopic examination will reveal colour, consistency and presence of haemoptysis.
- Material from lung abscess may be 'smelly'. In heart failure it is pink and frothy.
- Viscid sputum indicates presence of eosinophils and allergic stigmata.
- Special staining for aspergillus and pneumocystis, asbestos bodies.

Allergy tests
- Useful in diagnosis of asthma (extrinsic)

- Skin tests or 'RAST' available and especially useful in children.
- Helps to define treatment (disodium cromoglycate, Intal).
- Avoid allergen if possible.

Chest X-ray
- Ask for lateral
- Repeat if indicated

- Chest X-ray is mandatory in a smoker. Lateral film often useful especially in left lung lesions.
- If symptoms persist – repeat.

RESPIRATORY DISEASES

> *Lung function tests*
> - FEV$_1$, FVC, PEFR.
> - Transfer factor and lung volumes in a few.

- Needed to assess reversibility of airway obstruction – if present.
- A very low transfer factor may indicate fibrosis and emphysema.
- Repeat tests after treatment.
- Flow volume loops (*see below*) will distinguish upper/lower airway diseases.

> *ENT opinion*
> - When nasal and upper respiratory symptoms predominate

- Cough, rhinitis and stridor may suggest allergic and granulomatous disorders.
- Nasopharyngeal/laryngeal tumours to exclude.

> *Bronchoscopy*
> - Usually following specialist assessment

- Unresolved cough in a smoker with other symptoms – refer for a specialist opinion.

Types of cough

- Bronchial asthma

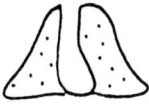
WHEEZE

- Dry, irritating, distressing at night. Exacerbated by exercise, emotion and cold air. Sputum – thick, 'stringy', 'glue'-like.

- Chronic bronchitis and emphysema

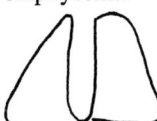
HYPERINFLATED CHEST

- Early morning 'rattle', sputum, easy to expectorate (mucopurulent).

- Bronchiectasis (cystic fibrosis lung abscess)

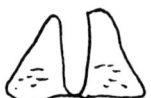
CRACKLES

- Cough all day and night. Large quantity of sputum.

SYMPTOMS AND THEIR MANAGEMENT

- Viral infections

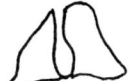
NO SIGNS

- Distressing cough but self-limiting (2–3 weeks). Very little sputum.

- Tuberculosis

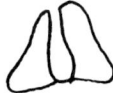
NO SIGNS IN EARLY DISEASE

- Paroxysmal cough with sputum, haemoptysis, weight loss, sweats.

- Lung cancer, pleurisy

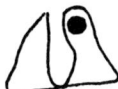
MONOPHONIC WHEEZE and PLEURAL RUB

- Prolonged, painful.

- Heart failure/alveolitis

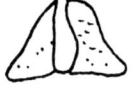
GENERALIZED CRACKLES

- A breathless patient with orthopnoea and PND, dry cough.

Management

- Two thirds of patients with significant respiratory conditions

- Most coughs have an organic basis.
- When part of common viral illness of upper/lower respiratory tract – only symptomatic treatment necessary.
- If there is evidence of more chronic respiratory disorders, then treat these.

Child: persistent cough
- Treat as asthma

- Most difficult problem in children with perennial nocturnal cough. If this is accompanied by wheeze and positive family history of allergy – then treat the child as asthmatic.

'Nerves'
- Do not dismiss – assess and explain

- Most patients and relatives dislike being told that the cough is due to 'nerves' especially when usually it is not! Sympathy, detailed examination ± chest X-ray will reassure most.

> *Cough suppressants*
> • Avoid if possible

• Many cough suppressants and expectorants are available. Often these may exacerbate the situation by causing drowsiness, respiratory depression and retention of sputum. Constipation is also a problem – as many contain codeine.

SORE THROAT

What is it?

Sore throats are very frequent – more than 100 episodes per GP per year.

• Who affected?

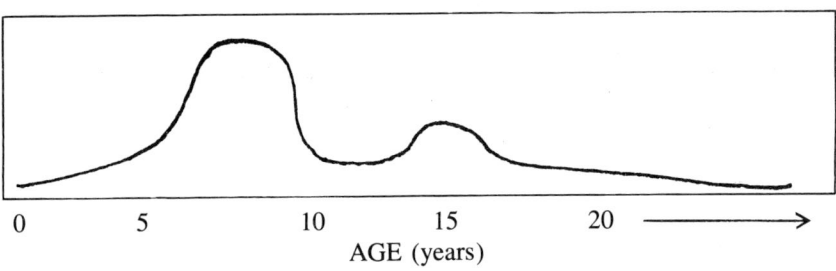

Two peaks of prevalence, at 4–8 and 15–20.

• Reasons for peaks are probable natural changes in immunology as they affect lymph tissues.

Causes and types

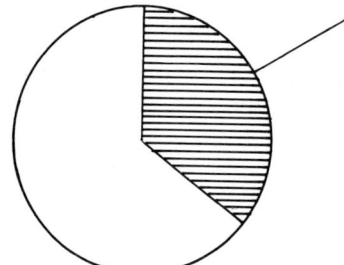

In only one third can specific pathogenic organisms be isolated,

i.e. β-Streptococci, pneumococci, *H. influenzae*

• *Note* glandular fever as a cause of sore throat at 15–20 years.
• Most acute sore throats are part of a more generalized upper respiratory infection.

- Serious types such as
    - diphtheria
    - quinsy
    - retropharyngeal abscess
    - epiglottitis

  are very rare.

Types – appearances

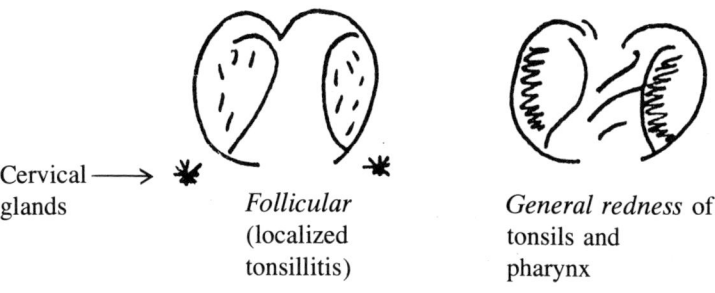

Cervical glands →

Follicular (localized tonsillitis)

General redness of tonsils and pharynx

- *Appearances* do not correlate with causes.
- *Importance*

  frequent

  most not caused by specific pathogens

  short period of sickness up to 1 week

  few complications
  - nephritis 1/2500
  - rheumatic fever 1/5000.

Aims of treatment

- Relieve symptoms
- Specific antibiotics?

Problems

- Appearances do not help in diagnosis of specific types.
- Self-limiting condition.
- Complications very rare.

- Should antibiotics be used, for what and which drug?
- Investigation – throat swabs have limited practical use. Blood test *only* to diagnose glandular fever (GF) in teenagers whose sore throats go on for more than a week.

Management

- *Explain* nature and likely cause of condition to patient and family.
- *Relieve symptoms* with analgesics (aspirin or paracetamol).
- *Antibiotics*
  Penicillin V
  Do not use ampicillin or amoxicillin – cause rashes in GF
  Erythromycin for penicillin sensitive.
- *Penicillin V*
  Intramuscular (Triplopen) for severe cases.
  Oral for up to 5 days (250 mg 4-hourly in adults).

CROUP

What is it?

- Acute inflammation of larynx and adjacent tissues caused by RSV, *Haemophilus influenzae* and other viruses.
- Who affected? Croup is almost confined to infants between 6 months and 3 years.
- Frightening for parents and distressing for child.
- Classical picture – child wakes at 11 p.m. to 2 a.m. with barking cough and some breathing difficulties.

Significance

- *Usually self-limiting* – once a child falls asleep symptoms improve and by morning well.
- *Acute upper respiratory obstruction* occurs in fewer than 1% – these require hospitalization.
- *Acute epiglottitis* may be confused – a very dangerous condition caused by *H. influenzae*. It can cause death by suffocation. Child very ill – little cough – cannot swallow – breathing difficult +++. Diagnosis must be made on probability – do not try and examine the throat, as it may tip balance into extreme laryngeal obstruction.

Management

- Reassure parents, the noisy cough and discomfort are not serious by themselves.
- Comfort the child.
- Advise – warm drinks, 'steam-kettle' in kitchen or in bathroom.
- Explain that once child goes to sleep the attack will pass and there is no need for parents to stay awake and observe.
- Beware of the one in 100 who is seriously distressed and who will benefit by admission to hospital for observation and reassurance.
- *Antibiotics* are not indicated.
- *Acute epiglottitis* – if suspected give i.m. injection of hydrocortisone 100 mg and take to a Paediatric Unit at once.

'FLU'

What is it?

Note the difference between *epidemic influenza* and endemic *'flu-like'* illnesses.

Epidemic influenza is devastating in its infectivity, causing large numbers of acutely ill persons within a short period – increasing practice work load ++.

Flu-like illnesses are caused by a variety of viral and bacterial pathogens with common features of sudden onset, aching, intense malaise, respiratory or gastrointestinal ('gastric flu') symptoms.

Significance

- High infectivity among patients and practice staff.
- Hospital admissions difficult because of blocked beds.
- Complications – respiratory, acute bronchitis, pneumonia and acute respiratory failure are most likely in respiratory invalids, elderly and infants.
- Case mortality is low; one per 1000 cases
- Most cases of influenza recover over 1–2 weeks, acute symptoms for 1 week followed by a period of debility.

Management

- *Acute attack*

(1) Advise:
    fluid diet
    analgesics

RESPIRATORY DISEASES

   (2)   Antibiotics should not be prescribed routinely but for specific reasons only
- *Complications*

   (1)   Bronchitis and pneumonia treat with antibiotics (which?)
   (2)   Respiratory failure requires urgent admission
- *Prophylaxis* – what value of immunization – highly questionable

COMMON URI (UPPER RESPIRATORY INFECTIONS – COUGHS, COLDS AND CATARRH)

What are they?

Inevitable and occur all over world
- Each person is likely to suffer 2–3 URI per year.
- *Age prevalence*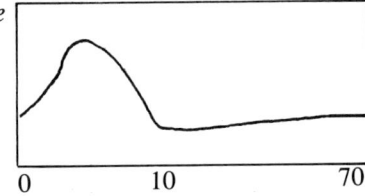
- Caused by viruses, but note that some 'colds' are nasal allergies.
- Course – '3 days coming, 3 days there and 3 days going'.

Significance

URI – a great nuisance.
- No complications likely in fit persons.
- Possible flare-up of chronic respiratory conditions.

Management

- *Explain* that no cures or prevention possible.
- *Symptomatic relief*
  hot drinks
  analgesic
  simple linctus
- *Antibiotics* not necessary unless complications as
  acute bronchitis/pneumonia
  acute sinusitis
  acute otitis media

WHEEZE

It is useful to relate this to the phase of respiration.

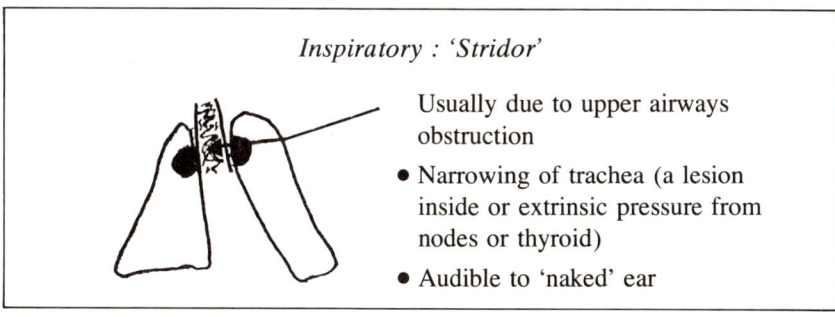

Inspiratory : 'Stridor'

Usually due to upper airways obstruction

- Narrowing of trachea (a lesion inside or extrinsic pressure from nodes or thyroid)
- Audible to 'naked' ear

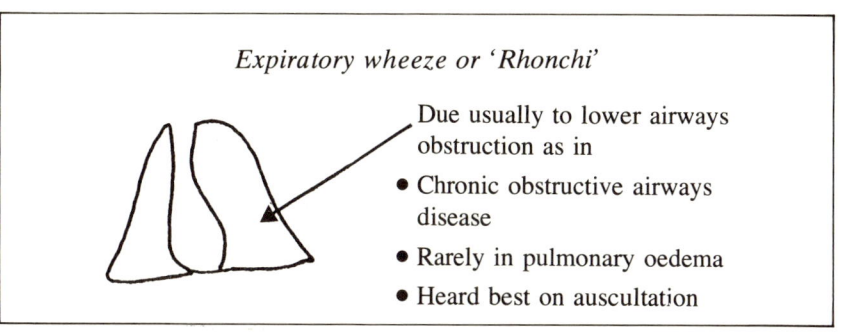

Expiratory wheeze or 'Rhonchi'

Due usually to lower airways obstruction as in

- Chronic obstructive airways disease
- Rarely in pulmonary oedema
- Heard best on auscultation

Monophonic wheeze

- Lesion in main or segmented bronchi, e.g. tumour, foreign body

Polyphonic wheeze

- Lesion in terminal bronchioles or alveoli: e.g. asthma, bronchitis

In cases of severe acute asthma the chest may sound 'quiet' as there is very little movement of air in the small airways. This can often mislead. Measurement of peak expiratory flow rate (PEFR) would help in this situation.

Stridor or inspiratory wheeze is audible in most cases, but in very mild upper airway obstruction the sign could be elicited by putting the stethoscope over the trachea.

Crackles are rarely heard in emphysema or asthma unless these conditions are complicated by infection or heart failure.

Causes of stridor

- Children
    croup
    epiglottitis
- Tracheal or laryngeal stenosis – following
    tracheostomy
    irradiation
    trauma
    tumour (benign and malignant)
- Arterial aneurysm
- Thyroid and thymus enlargement
- Dermoid cysts
- Tetanus
- Lymph nodes secondary to cancer, leukaemia, Hodgkin's and sarcoid
- Lesions in the pharynx or oesophagus

Management

Detailed examination of the patient may reveal the cause:

1. *Stridor*	
Test	*Possible findings*
• Chest X-ray	• May be normal or show upper mediastinal enlargement or shadow
• Blood tests	• Very high ESR may indicate neoplasm or Hodgkin's
	• Abnormality of thyroid function
• Scanning	• Relevant thyroid abnormality, e.g. multinodular goitre

Whom to refer for specialist opinion?

When symptoms and signs persist and above tests are normal, the patient should be referred to ear, nose, throat or chest specialist. Laryngoscopy, oesophagoscopy, bronchoscopy and possibly mediastinoscopy may be necessary.

- Fibreoptic bronchoscopy may be very hazardous for the patient in presence of stridor.

2. Monophonic wheeze	
Test	*Possible findings*
• Chest X-ray (a lateral is useful)	• Ill-defined opacity suggesting bronchial carcinoma, carcinoid tumour or bronchopneumonia. Distal collapse of lung may result from a foreign body, sputum plugging, caseation due to TB and granuloma
• Blood tests	• Anaemia, leukocytosis, eosinophilia and high ESR may give a clue to the underlying diagnosis
• Sputa	• Malignant cells or acid fast bacilli

3. Polyphonic wheeze	
Test	*Possible findings*
• Chest X-ray	• May be normal. Hyperinflation will suggest airways obstruction due to emphysema, bronchitis, asthma and bronchiectasis
• Blood tests	• High haemoglobin may indicate secondary polycythaemia. Eosinophilia may indicate asthma (Note a very high eosinophil count and ESR due to polyarteritis nodosa and eosinophilic granuloma)

Who to refer to hospital?

- Most patients with persistent monophonic wheeze will need a firm diagnosis. Bronchoscopy may be necessary.
- Patients with polyphonic wheezes could turn out to have chronic obstructive airways disorders. Specialist help is only necessary if results of tests are misleading or in those who do not respond to therapy.
- Unlike cough which can exist without any other accompanying respiratory symptoms, wheeze is usually associated with other symptoms that can help in the diagnosis. Respiratory function tests are helpful in distinguishing the cause or source of the wheeze. In a smoking wheezy patient a peak expiratory flow rate (PEFR) of less than 200 l/min and ratio of forced expiratory volume (FEV_1) to forced vital capacity (FVC) of less than 50% may indicate chronic bronchitis and emphysema. A higher variable result of PEFR would indicate bronchial asthma. When PEFR rises by over 20% after a bronchodilator (200 μg of salbutamol or 0.16 mg of isoprenaline) then the diagnosis of asthma should be strongly considered. *Flow volume loops (see below)* are invaluable in distinguishing not only upper from lower respiratory disorders but also the different chronic obstructive airways disorders.

Flow volume loops

- Majority of lung function laboratories undertake the test.
- Make a special request for it.
- Indicate why.
- A useful adjuvant to 'basic' tests of lung function.

Special indications

- To define whether mainly obstruction or restriction of airways.
- What type of obstruction { upper respiratory. lower respiratory.

Types

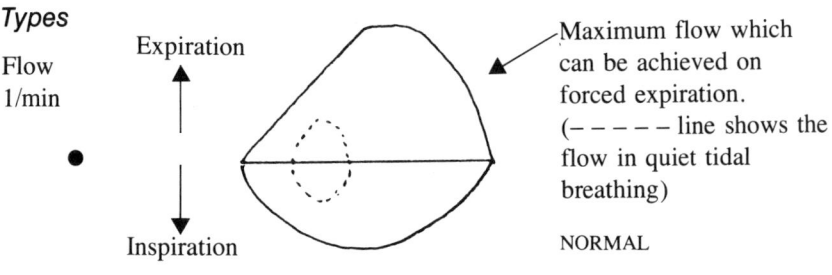

Flow l/min

Expiration
Inspiration

Maximum flow which can be achieved on forced expiration.
(— — — — — line shows the flow in quiet tidal breathing)

NORMAL

Flow
l/min

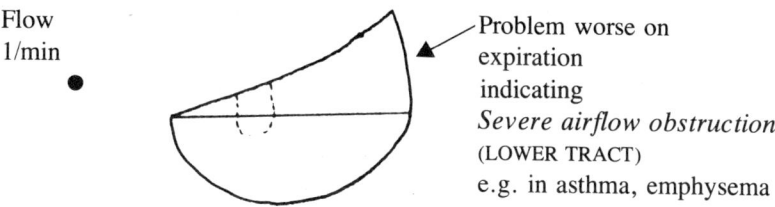

Problem worse on expiration indicating
Severe airflow obstruction
(LOWER TRACT)
e.g. in asthma, emphysema

Flow
l/min

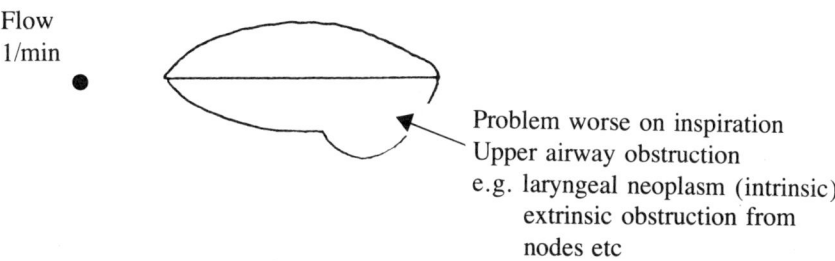

Problem worse on inspiration
Upper airway obstruction
e.g. laryngeal neoplasm (intrinsic)
extrinsic obstruction from nodes etc

	A wheezy child
Disorder	*Likely type of wheeze* (M) *Monophonic* (P) *Polyphonic*
Bronchial asthma	(P)
Respiratory infections (viral and bacterial)	(P)
Inhalation of foreign body	(M)
Bronchiectasis (including cystic fibrosis)	(M) and (P)

A wheezy adult	
Disorder	Likely type of wheeze (M) *Monophonic* (P) *Polyphonic*
Bronchial asthma	(P)
Bronchitis	(M) and (P)
Bronchiectasis	(M) and (P)
Carcinoma of lung	(M)
TB and sarcoidosis	(M)

BREATHLESSNESS

Normally an individual breathes at a rate of 14–18 per minute and is unaware of the effort. Dyspnoea or breathlessness is present when the patient is aware of this and especially if he or she experiences discomfort. The problem may be extrapulmonary.

Cardiovascular
- Heart failure
- Pericarditis
- Cardiomyopathy
- Left ventricular failure due to
    (1) high blood pressure
    (2) ischaemic heart disease

Musculoskeletal/Nervous system
- Ankylosing spondylitis
- Kyphoscoliosis
- Myasthenia gravis
- Ascending polyneuritis
- Mononeuritis multiplex

> *Miscellaneous*
> - Pregnancy
> - Thyrotoxicosis
> - Anaemia

Constant dyspnoea

This is a feature of chronic lung disorders such as bronchitis, emphysema, bronchiectasis, fibrosing and allergic alveolitis. Paroxysmal dyspnoea with wheeze will occur in bronchial asthma. Acute or recently developed dyspnoea may be secondary to infection including pneumonia, pulmonary oedema, pleurisy, pleural effusion, pulmonary embolism and pneumothorax.

Disproportionate dyspnoea[1]

This is also known as *psychogenic dyspnoea*

- The diagnosis should be made only when other significant lung diseases have been excluded.
- The patient would describe difficulty in breathing at rest. 'Vivid' terms would be used, e.g. 'cannot get enough air in', 'can't fill my lungs properly' etc.
- The patient is worse in stressful situations.
- Exercise in the early stages may cause tachycardia – later patient is able to 'cope' quite well.
- It is not a 'common' problem.

> *Psychogenic or disproportionate dyspnoea*
> - Well recognized
> - Occurs in anxious individuals
> - Tendency to panic
> - Men = females
> - Increase respiratory rate, tachycardia, paraesthesiae, cold, sweaty hands
> - Arterial blood gases show normal P_{O_2} and low P_{CO_2} ± metabolic acidosis (respiratory alkalosis)
> - Patient often unaware of the problem
> - Explain, strong reassurance necessary

Common causes of acute nocturnal dyspnoea

- Left ventricular failure
- Pulmonary embolism
- Bronchial asthma

Left ventricular failure

- Background of hypertension or ischaemic heart disease
- May be accompanied by chest pain
- Patient crouching forward, cold and clammy
- Poor volume, fast pulse
- Crackles at bases of lungs
- Give diuretics, diamorphine $\pm$ aminophylline, digoxin
- Hospital admission may be necessary

Pulmonary embolism

- Patient often obese, immobile, smoking and female
- Taking contraceptive 'pill'
- Positive previous and family history
- Cold, clammy, cyanosed, in pain
- Pleural rub or effusion
- Analgesics, oxygen (if available) – hospital admission for heparin and anticoagulants

---

Bronchial asthma

- In many, previous history of asthma and allergy to house dust mite
- Preceding infection
- Patient crouching forward, fast pulse with paradox. Warm peripheries
- Confusion and aggression due to anoxia
- Give reassurance, oxygen (if available), aminophylline (*slowly*) (i.v.) and hydrocortisone (i.v.)
- May need to be hospitalized even when there is early improvement. Patients often need constant assessment for 7–10 days after an attack.

CHEST PAIN

> *Cardiac ischaemia*
>
> - The retrosternal 'heavy' 'band-like' chest discomfort and pain radiating down the arms, towards the back and the jaw is suggestive of cardiac ischaemia
> - A chest X-ray may be necessary to exclude a lung abnormality. It may also show enlargement of heart
> - Electrocardiograph (including in some cases stress e.c.g) is mandatory
> - Specialist assessment is necessary in many 'young' patients

> *Pain of respiratory disorders*
>
> - 'Nagging', localized discomfort (persistent) – may indicate bronchogenic carcinoma
> - 'Sharp-shooting' pleuritic pain – as a result of pleurisy, rib fractures, pneumonia, pneumothorax, pulmonary infarction and splenic/liver disorders
> - 'Tightness' – bronchial asthma, fibrosis
> - Generalized, one-sided 'heavy' pain – mesothelioma, post-thoracotomy or pneumonectomy, emphysema or abscess
> - A chest X-ray (PA and lateral film) necessary
> - Many will need further specialist care

HAEMOPTYSIS

Streaking of sputum with blood or its products must be taken seriously as it often signifies disease. However, in about 10–15% of patients no cause for bleeding is found even after exhaustive investigations. Bronchiectasis used to be regarded as the commonest cause of painless haemoptysis. Bronchiectasis would produce large quantities of purulent sputum as well. Currently bronchogenic carcinoma and pulmonary infarction have surpassed bronchiectasis as the main cause. The haemoptysis in bronchogenic carcinoma is usually accompanied by some degree of pain.

Common causes of haemoptysis

Painless
- Bronchiectasis (usually large quantities of mucopurulent sputum)
- Pulmonary oedema
- Tuberculosis

Painful
- Bronchogenic carcinoma
- Pulmonary embolism and infarction
- Pneumonia
- Trauma ± rib fracture

Management

Ask the patient

(1) Quantity and quality of sputum and blood expectorated?
(2) Previous history of relevance?
(3) Possibility of aspiration?
(4) How long?
(5) Vomiting or dyspepsia?
(6) 'Pill'?

Investigations

Chest X-ray in haemoptysis

- This is necessary in all patients with haemoptysis
- If no abnormality reported and the haemoptysis persists, then a further film with a lateral film may help
- If doubt about the 'hilar shadows' – ask for tomograms

Sputa tests in haemoptysis

- Microscopy and culture for bacteria, fungi and acid-fast bacilli. Special staining necessary for fungi. Three specimens (separate) useful if TB suspected.
- Cytology for malignant cells. False negatives few – therefore a useful test

---

Who to refer for specialist opinion?

- Any smoker who has one or two episodes of haemoptysis, especially with doubtful chest film and sputa cytology.
- A young non-smoker with persistent haemoptysis may have bronchiectasis or carcinoid tumour (benign)/bronchial adenoma. A chest X-ray may often be normal.
- Any history of inhalation of a foreign body, especially a peanut. In a child it may result in pneumonia.
- A miner with persistent haemoptysis (especially 'tarry' material) may indicate development of progressive massive fibrosis, TB, or cancer. A patient with pneumoconiosis will eventually need 'panel' assessment regarding compensation.
- In haemosiderosis and chronic pulmonary oedema, assessment of underlying cardiac disorder, e.g. mitral stenosis, is necessary. In these cases the chest X-ray may already have shown a 'globular' heart as well as widespread calcified and nodular shadowing.
- If pulmonary embolism is likely in a 'pill'-taking young female – treatment will be in hospital. A ventilation/perfusion lung scan is necessary. A decision regarding duration of anticoagulants and future contraception should be between the specialist and general practitioner.

	Child with haemoptysis
Persistent	• Cystic fibrosis/bronchiectasis
	• Foreign body
Acute	• Prolonged coughing as in acute bronchitis, asthma
	• Trauma

	Young adult with haemoptysis
Smoker	• Bronchogenic cancer (early)
	• Acute and chronic bronchitis
	• Bronchiectasis
Non-smoker	• Bronchial adenoma
	• Pulmonary embolism
	• Mitral stenosis
	• Bronchiectasis
	• Tuberculosis

RESPIRATORY DISEASES

	Middle-aged person with haemoptysis
Smoker ♂ ≥ ♀	• Bronchogenic carcinoma • Bronchiectasis
Non-smoker	• Bronchiectasis • Acute lower respiratory tract infection • Tuberculosis

	Old person with haemoptysis
Smoker *or* *a non-smoker*	• Bronchogenic cancer • Tuberculosis • Bronchiectasis • Recurrent aspiration pneumonia, e.g. paraffin, achalasia

Reference

1   Editorial. (1981). Hyperventilation and anxiety state. *J. Roy. Soc. Med.*, **74**, 1

CASE HISTORIES

Case 1

A 55-year old man has had – over 3 months – 'dry' cough, breathlessness, slight chest pain and weight loss > 6 kg. He is a smoker.

• Examination is normal
    Chest X-ray shows a probable lesion in the left lower lobe.

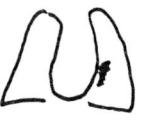

• Referred to a specialist.
    FEV_1 (forced expiratory volume) is greater than 1.8 litres.
    Sputum and blood tests normal.
    Bronchoscopy revealed *a squamous cell carcinoma* of apical segment of left lower lobe.
    Liver/bone scan normal. Left lower lobectomy. No major complications. Patient alive, with no evidence of secondaries 2 years later.

Case 2

A 25-year-old white woman (non-smoker) has a 'dry' cough, slight retrosternal

discomfort and breathlessness. Describes red, raised nodules over the front of the legs. No eye or 'joints' trouble.
- Examination confirms erythema nodosum. No nodal, liver or spleen enlargement.
- A diagnosis of *sarcoidosis* made.
- Chest X-ray shows bilateral hilar enlargement and a right paratracheal node.

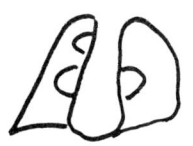

- Diagnosis was explained to the patient. Aspirin/paracetamol suggested. Reviewed at 4 weeks. No signs or symptoms. Asked to return if recurrence of symptoms. Chest X-ray repeated at 6 months, 12 months and 2 years.

Case 3

A child has quite severe cough and wheeze during spring/summer months. Positive history of 'allergy'.
- Examination: 'nasal' speech, eczema (flexural), polyphonic wheeze in both lung fields.
- Diagnosis of *asthma/eczema/hay fever* made.
- Referred for advice on treatment including desensitization.

Case 4

A 55-year-old smoking chronic bronchitic with constant dyspnoea develops acute illness of cough, fever, 'green' sputum, profuse sweating and drowsiness.
- Examination: possible right lower lobe pneumonia ? post-influenzal.
- Admitted to hospital urgently. Respiratory failure P_{CO_2} ↑ P_{O_2} ↓ confirmed. Chest X-ray showed *right middle and lower lobe pneumonia*.

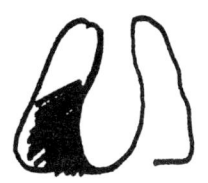

Given antibiotics, oxygen, physiotherapy and improved.

Case 5

A young child suddenly has distressing cough followed by dyspnoea ± stridor. GP is urgently summoned – acute respiratory distress diagnosed – patient escorted to hospital (oxygen and facility to intubate/tracheotomy).

- Chest X-ray: collapse of right middle/lower lobe

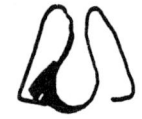

  left lung clear

- Inhalation of foreign body likely, removed on bronchoscopy. The child made full recovery.

Case 6

A 60-year-old man (non-smoker) admits TB (treated) previously and now has cough productive of large quantities of sputum (1 cupful a day) with haemoptysis.

- Examination: finger clubbing and basal crackles.
- Chest X-ray: diffuse reticular/cavitating shadowing at the bases and left apex

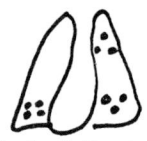

- Referred to a specialist with the following possibilities:

   post-TB bronchiectasis
   aspergillosis and other allergy disorders
   reactivation of TB
   fibrocystic disease.

Tests including bronchogram confirm *severe bilateral bronchiectasis*. Postural drainage and antibiotics failed to control the disease and patient died in respiratory failure.

Case 7

An anxious 40-year-old man suddenly develops severe lower chest pain (tightness) following mild viral illness.

- Examination reveals distress, sweating, tenderness on palpation of right lower chest and abdomen.
- Referred to hospital. Chest X-ray, e.c.g. normal.
- *Viral pleurisy or Börnholm disease* diagnosed; responded to reassurance and indomethacin.

Case 8

A 44-year-old smoking man presented with 'noisy' breathlessness and slight discomfort in the throat.

- Examination revealed stridor (inspiratory wheeze).
- Chest X-ray was normal.
- Referred to a specialist. A diagnosis of upper respiratory tract obstruction made. Flow volume loops confirmed this. Laryngoscopy/bronchoscopy showed a *laryngeal tumour* (operable). No lung involvement.

Case 9

An 18-year-old woman (non-smoker) has dry, irritating cough with wheeze especially on exercise and at night. Family history of 'allergy'.

- Examination: polyphonic wheezes (a few) in the chest.
- PEFR (peak expiratory flow rate) = 300 l/min. (Predicted = 450 l/min.)
- A diagnosis of *extrinsic asthma* made. Diagnosis explained and advice on avoiding common allergies – house dust/mite.
- Prescribed beclomethasone aerosol inhalers to be taken twice a day for 3 months and salbutamol or terbutaline or ipratropium when necessary.

    Inhaler technique supervised.

    Review at 2 weeks: improvement. PEFR 400 l/min. Mouth clear of candida (side-effect in some of steroid inhalers). Treatment continued. At 3 months – 'steroid' inhaler stopped and advised to take again during exacerbation.

Case 10

A 47-year-old *late onset asthmatic* – on steroids (prednisone) for 10 years – is *concerned* about continuing on therapy especially as she 'needs' 10 mg/day. On maximum oral and inhaled therapy.

- Specialist opinion sought regarding 'nebulizer' therapy and any other 'alternatives' to long-term steroids.
- Nebulizer recommended. Parenteral (i.m.) triamcinolone 80 mg tried every 4 – 6 weeks. Synacthen test shows a good response and therefore able to reduce prednisone to 2 mg/day over 3 months. Continuing supervision, prednisone then stopped and nebulizer (at least twice a day) and triamcinolone maintained. A further 10-day course of prednisone and antibiotics necessary for acute infective exacerbation. Triamcinolone stopped after 9 months and then given SOS. During this period no major side-effects of triamcinolone, e.g. proximal muscle wasting, bruising or hair loss occurred. Patient remained under GP-hospital care.

RESPIRATORY DISEASES

Case 11

A 68-year-old non-smoker complains of cough and 'wheeze' especially at night. Breathless on 'shopping'. Previously healthy.

- Examination, electrocardiograph normal.
- PEFR 260 1/min. Chest X-ray

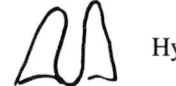

  Hyperinflation

- Diagnosis of *late onset intrinsic asthma* made.
- Patient's aerosol inhaler technique poor. Haler-aid (Allen & Hanbury), Spacer also of no help. Slow-release preparations of salbutamol, terbutaline and theophylline not tolerated. Patient stops treatment. On review, PEFR reduced to 160 1/min – worsening wheeze and cough at night.
- Prednisone 45 mg/day for 3 days, 30 mg/day for 3 days and then 20 mg/day prescribed. Told to report back in 24 h if no better. Specialist referral sent asking:

    (1) ? is the current treatment appropriate;
    (2) ? any further suggestions;
    (3) ? plan for long-term therapy
        ? steroids
        ? nebulizer;
    (4) ? clinic (hospital) supervision.

- On review in 10 days: patient very much better. PEFR 360 1/min. Mild indigestion – enteric-coated preparation used. Maintained on 10 mg/day.

Case 12

A 50-year-old smoking man has cough, breathlessness, painful ankles and weight loss.

- Examination reveals a left pleural effusion ?? collapse; gynaecomastia, tender 'hot' ankles.
- A probable diagnosis of *lung cancer*.
- Referred to specialist (urgent).
  Chest X-ray showed collapse of left lower lobe.

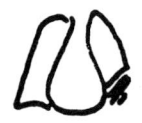

Long bones (X-rays) show features of HPOA (hypertrophic pulmonary osteoarthropathy).

Bronchoscopy revealed a left main bronchus squamous cell carcinoma. Not operable.

Patient's cough, breathlessness and HPOA responded to radiotherapy but he died 6 months later.

Case 13

A 58-year-old smoking man admits to cough and sputum for 3 months in a year (winter) for the past 2–3 years.

- Examination: a heavy, slightly cyanosed man with nicotine-stained fingers. PEFR less than 180 l/min. Chest X-ray shows severe hyperinflation.

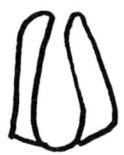

- A diagnosis of *chronic bronchitis and emphysema* is made. Fails to give up smoking as advised. No significant benefit from salbutamol or theophylline preparations. Antibiotics: repeated courses.
- A year later develops ankle swelling and further reduction in exercise tolerance. *Cor pulmonale* diagnosed. Diuretics prescribed. PEFR 110 l/min.
- Referred to a specialist:
  (1) ? oxygen
  (2) ? steroids
  (3) ? longer courses of antibiotics
  (4) ? physiotherapy
  (5) ? supervision in hospital
- Patient fails to respond to any form of therapy – confined to home and dies 4 years later.

Case 14

A 70-year-old smoking man has cough, productive of sputum and intermittent haemoptysis for 18 months. Marked breathlessness, weight loss and chest pain.
- Examination reveals a cachetic man with finger clubbing, large right-sided pleural effusion, hepatomegaly and supraclavicular nodes.
- Diagnosis of *disseminated malignancy* made.

RESPIRATORY DISEASES

- The patient lives alone. Domiciliary chest X-ray confirms pleural effusion and contralateral lung secondaries.

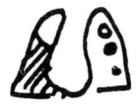

Hospice care team involved. Patient died peacefully in a hospice within 3 weeks.

Case 15

A 3-year-old child has cough and wheeze, especially at night and during winter months. No history of allergy. Family 'smoke'.

- Examination normal.
- Diagnosis of *chronic wheezy bronchitis*.
- Dangers to the child from parents' smoke explained. Reassured that 'it' will improve as the child gets older. Specialist help not necessary here. Mild theophylline elixir at night was prescribed and was regarded as beneficial.

Case 16

A 50-year-old man presents with progressive dyspnoea, cough, orthopnoea and limitation of exercise tolerance. He had stopped smoking 10 years previously. Admits to asbestos exposure over a 16-year period (before 1974).

- Examination: finger clubbing, cyanosis and basal lung crackles.
- Referred for assessment:

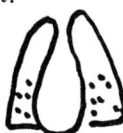

Chest X-ray — increased basal reticulation

- A diagnosis of *fibrosing alveolitis* probably due to asbestosis. Histological confirmation.
- Patient made aware of diagnosis. Case notified. Compensation procedure if appropriate. Condition deteriorated in spite of continuous oxygen and patient died in respiratory/heart failure.

Case 17

A 28-year-old smoking mother of two children develops left lower pleuritic chest pain with dizziness, slight haemoptysis and breathlessness. She is on 'the pill'.

- Examination: ? pleural rub at the left base. Tenderness on palpation of left calf.

- A diagnosis of *pulmonary infarction/leg thrombosis*.
- Chest X-ray: normal.
- Referred to hospital. 'Pill' stopped. Lung scan positive. Advised not to take the 'pill' again. GP was informed and asked to refer to Family Planning Unit if necessary. On anticoagulants for 3 months.

Case 18

A 37-year-old asthmatic on non-steroidal inhalation only develops cough, fever, sweats, 'plugs' of yellow sputum and weight loss.

- Examination: ill-looking, pale person.
- Referred for assessment:

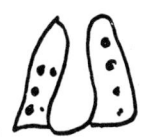

'patchy' peripheral pneumonitis

high ESR and eosinophil count, aspergillus skin reaction and precipitins were positive.

- Diagnosis of *bronchopulmonary aspergillosis* made. Patient responded rapidly to steroids.

Case 19

A healthy 30-year-old non-smoking man has cough and recurrent slight haemoptysis.

- Examination and chest X-ray normal.
- Referred to a specialist. Bronchoscopy revealed an operable *bronchial adenoma*.

Case 20

A farmer develops acute cough and wheeze – after a weekend 'break'.

- Examination: crackles over the upper zones.
- Possible diagnosis of 'allergy'.
- Referred for assessment:

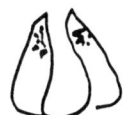

    Chest X-ray   Upper zone opacity
Negative tests for TB.

- Diagnosis of *allergic alveolitis* made. Very good response to prednisone. Change of job advised. Patient accepted this.

RESPIRATORY DISEASES

Case 21

A 45-year-old smoking woman has cough, sputum, haemoptysis, sweats, weight loss. Admits to excess alcohol. Previous TB 'scar' on the chest X-ray.

- Examination: ill woman. Palmar erythema, hepatomegaly and crackles over the upper zones of the lungs.
- A diagnosis of *reactivated pulmonary tuberculosis*.
- Chest X-ray

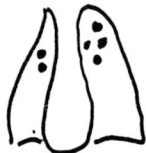

  bilateral cavitating upper lobe lesions
  Sputa + ve for AAFB (human)

- Urgent hospital treatment (isolation unit):

    notified to community physicians: contact tracing;
    help given to withdrawal of alcohol;

    careful monitor of eyes and liver: drugs used ethambutol, isoniazid, rifampicin and pyridoxine.

    Responded: sputa negative in 6 weeks. Chest X-ray clearing in 3 months.

Case 22

A previously healthy non-smoking young man presents with 'sharp' pleuritic chest pain followed by breathlessness (mild) and cough.

- Examination normal.
- A diagnosis of viral infection ? pleurisy ? pneumothorax.
- Chest X-ray

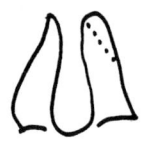

  a small left-sided *spontaneous pneumothorax;* less than 15% collapse

- Diagnosis explained to patient – 'kept at home' – advised on breathing exercises ± physiotherapy. A chest X-ray 36 h later shows complete resolution. (A further film only if recurrence/persistence of symptoms.)

Case 23

A 35-year-old man has 'flu' and then develops severe retrosternal tightness, sweating, palpitations.

- Examination: distress, ? pericardial friction rub.

- A diagnosis of *pericarditis* made. Electrocardiogram showed ST elevation and arrhythmia.
- Urgent hospital admission – responded to non-steroidal anti-inflammatory agents. Disopyramide was necessary for the arrhythmia – continued for 3 months. Patient made 'full' recovery.

Case 24

A 30-year-old woman who had recently delivered a baby became ill with breathlessness and haemoptysis.

- Referred immediately to hospital.
- Chest X-ray — widespread lesions
- Gynaecologist consulted. A diagnosis of *disseminated choriocarinoma* made and patient referred to specialist oncology unit.

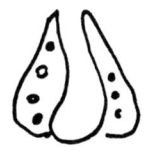

3

Radiological investigations

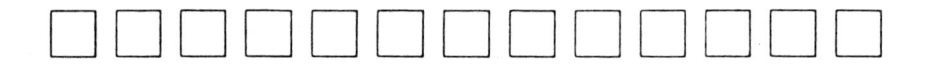

SIGNIFICANCE

This chapter deals mainly with the chest X-ray, the help it offers in diagnosing and managing respiratory disorders. The more complex investigations, e.g. tomography, bronchogram, lung-scan imaging and CAT scanning, may be necessary but it would be fair to suggest that these should be undertaken after a specialist assessment. Most general practitioners have open access to radiology departments and routine chest X-ray is a recognized essential in evaluating a clinical problem. On its own a chest X-ray could be misleading and therefore a clinical history and examination of the patient is necessary in all cases.

PROBLEMS

The common respiratory disorders, e.g. chronic bronchitis, emphysema, asthma and bronchiectasis, may produce no recognizable abnormality on the film. Even cases of lung cancer, especially if the lesion is small and occupying a large bronchus, may not be seen on the film. Only a minority (about 25%) of pulmonary embolism/infarction and pleural plaques will produce an abnormality on the film.

> *Normal chest X-ray in majority*
> - Chronic bronchitis or emphysema
> - Bronchial asthma
> - Early lung cancer and fibrosing alveolitis
> - Bronchial adenoma
> - Pulmonary embolism
> - Endobronchial granuloma

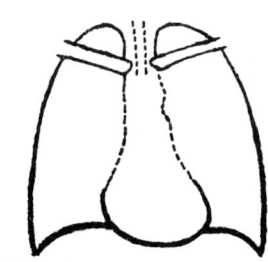

If an abnormality is noted on the film, enquiry should be made as regards any previous film and, if available, a comparison should be made for any changes.

> *Indications for a chest X-ray in general practice*
> - Sudden onset of dyspnoea, including stridor
> - Sudden onset of chest pain
> - Persisting breathlessness, chest pain, cough and sputum
> - Haemoptysis (especially in smokers)
> - Trauma to the chest
>   > Rib fractures, although clinically suspected, may not show on the film. If necessary to prove diagnosis – medicolegal reason – repeat the film in about 6 weeks.
> - Unexplained weight loss, night sweats, general malaise and PUO

COMMON ABNORMALITIES

Only the common findings are discussed. The reader is referred to a specialized text (Simon, G. (1978). 4th Edn. *Principles of Chest X-ray Diagnosis*. (London: Butterworth)) for further reading. It is useful to classify abnormalities under the following headings.

- Bony structure
- Heart shadow
- Soft tissues and miscellaneous shadows
- Hilar shadows
- Lung fields
- Pleural, pericardial, mediastinal and diaphragmatic abnormalities
- Abnormalities produced on the film by liver, spleen, ascites and upper gastrointestinal pathology.

Bony structure

> *Bony lesions seen on the chest X-ray*
>
> - Rib or thoracic spine fractures
> - Pathological fractures due to secondary deposits, osteoporosis, osteomalacia – detailed assessment necessary
>
> - Severe injury
> - Flail chest – refer to hospital
>
> - Kyphosis/scoliosis
> - May be congenital – no action if symptom-free
>
> - Cervical rib
> - Unilateral – relatively common. May cause 'pressure' symptoms. ? Surgical opinion
>
> - Infection
> - Soft tissue shadowing:
>   actinomycoses
>   osteomyelitis
>
> - Rib notching
> - In coarctation and neurofibromatosis

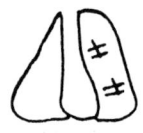

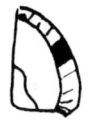

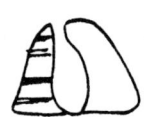

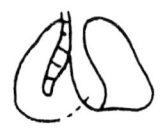

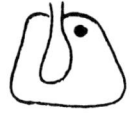

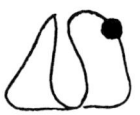

Abnormalities of heart shadow

Straight left heart border

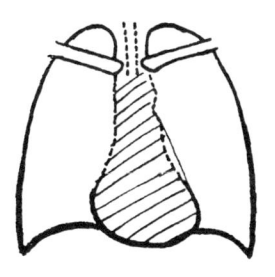

- Early left heart enlargement and failure
- Collapse of segments of left lower lobe

Globular shadow

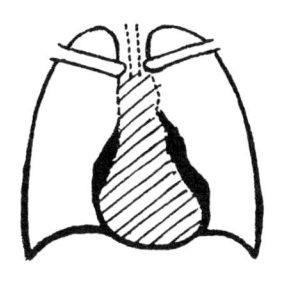

- Congestive cardiomyopathy
- Congestive heart failure
- Mitral valve disease

Wide-based heart (flower-vase abnormality)

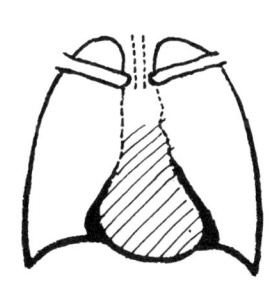

- Pericardial effusion
- Pericardial cyst

Causes of pericardial effusion
- Tamponade
- Myxoedema
- Acromegaly

Soft tissues and miscellaneous shadows

- Nipple shadows 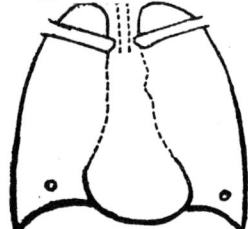
  - These could be confusing and may be reported as small nodules. A marker over the nipple will distinguish.

- Hair plaits 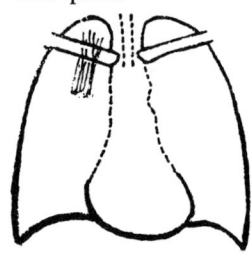
  - Especially in Indian women may be described as upper zone shadowing

- Missing breast shadow 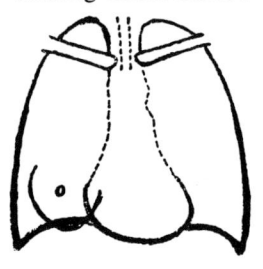
  - ? Mastectomy 2° to cancer

- Gynaecomastia 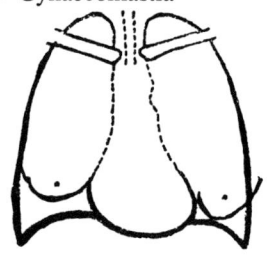
  - Pubertal
  - Cancer
  - Liver disorders
  - Drugs

- Valve prosthesis
  Central lines
  Pacing wires

Hilar shadows

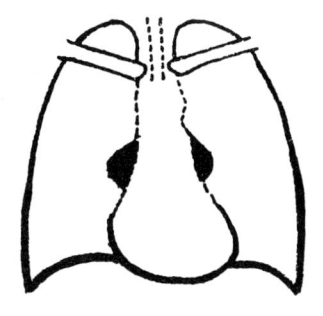

- Well defined due to prominent pulmonary vessels as in 2° pulmonary hypertension.
  Previous history of chronic airways obstruction

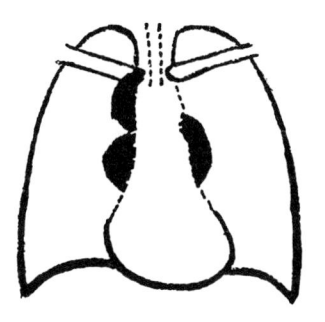

- Hilar glandular enlargement with para-tracheal shadow.
  TB
  Sarcoid
  Hodgkin's

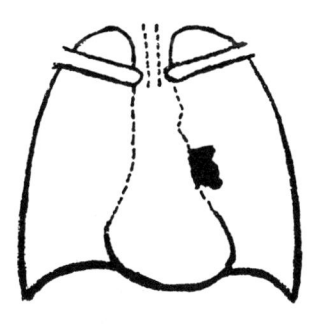

- Irregular shadow usually due to lung cancer

TOMOGRAPHY HELPFUL

Lung fields

Collapse of whole or part (lateral film very useful) suggested by:

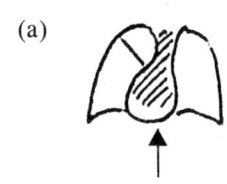

(a) Displaced transverse fissure
Right lateral necessary to define the segment of RUL collapsed
- endobronchial lesion

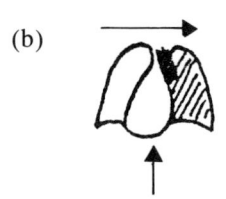

(b) Complete collapse of (L) lung with trachea deviated towards it
e.g. in carcinoma

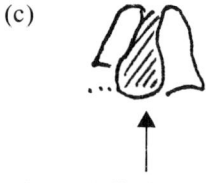

(c) Elevated diaphragm

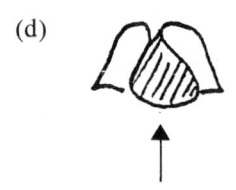

(d) Straight left heart border
- collapse of part of left lower lobe

Consolidation: There is usually some degree of collapse as well:

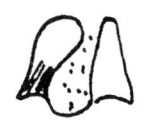

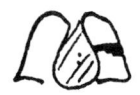

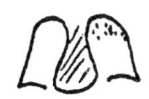

(a) *Consolidation of right lower lobe*
(if heart shadow visible RLL; if not, RML)
- bacterial pneumonias

(b) *Lingular consolidation*
(Lateral necessary)
- seen in 'atypical' pneumonias

(c) *Upper lobe consolidation*
Unilateral or bilateral
± cavities
- as in tuberculosis: aspergillosis

RADIOLOGICAL INVESTIGATIONS

Widespread shadowing

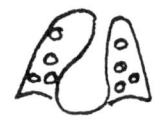

(a) Multiple rounded shadow as in
- secondary neoplasm
- Caplan's nodules

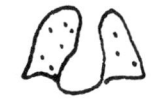

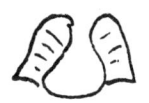

(b) Miliary ± calcification
- TB
- Chickenpox pneumonia
- mitral stenosis

(c) Large heart + increase in background shadowing
- heart failure

Basal shadowing

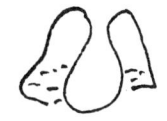

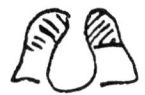

Increased reticulation: unilateral/bilateral
- fibrosis (cryptogenic)
- Kerley B lines in left heart failure
- alveolar carcinoma

Apical shadowing

Increased reticulation: mainly upper zones
- fibrosis (allergic)
- heart failure
- TB
- ankylosing spondylitis

Cavities/abscess

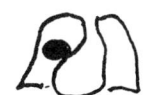

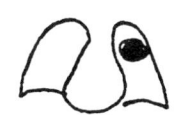

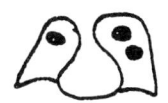

(a) Hilar/central
- cavitating squamous lung cancer
- rarely benign tumour

(b) Peripheral lesion
- TB
- aspergillus
- bacterial
- infected infarct

(c) Bilateral/multiple
- TB

RESPIRATORY DISEASES

'Coin' lesion

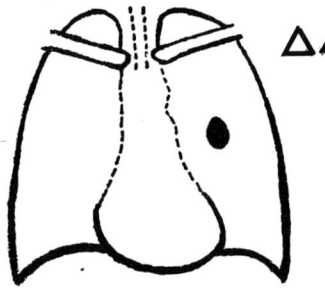

△△ • new growth (irregular margins)
- TB (tuberculoma with calcifications)
- pulmonary infarct
- single second primary or secondary
- cyst
- benign tumour, e.g. dermoid, haematoma
- AV malformation

Ask for tomogram

Pleural, pericardial, mediastinal and diaphragmatic abnormalities

Pleural

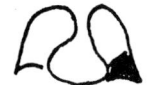

(a) Pleural effusion (unilateral/bilateral)
- new growth
- pneumonia
- pulmonary embolism/infarction
- TB
- collagen disease
- pancreatitis (L-sided)

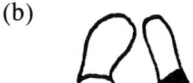

(b) Thickening (basal or apical)
- previous pleurisy
- chronic inflammatory disease, e.g. bronchitis

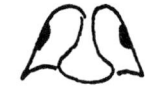

(c) Plaques ? calcified (special tangential views useful)
- asbestos
- TB (previous)

Types of fluid accumulated:

(1) Serous | transudate
            | exudate

(2) Blood: haemothorax (injury)

(3) Lymph: chylothorax (injury, cancer, leukaemia)

(4) Pus: empyema

RADIOLOGICAL INVESTIGATIONS

Pericardial

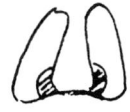

(a) Pad of fat
- of no significance
- could mislead
- ask for lateral and tomogram

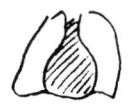

(b) Narrow neck
wide-base
'vase' appearance
Echo cardiogram necessary
- pericardial effusion
- tamponade

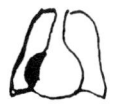

(c) Large cyst
- 'clear-water' Echocardiogram necessary

Mediastinal

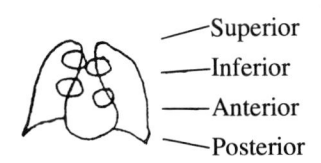

Superior
Inferior
Anterior
Posterior

Nodes (lymph)
cancer
sarcoid
Hodgkin's/leukaemia

Vascular
aortic dilatation

Glandular
thyroid (superior)
thymus (anterior)

Benign tumours
teratoma
dermoid cysts
lipoma

RESPIRATORY DISEASES

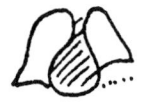

Diaphragmatic

(a) *Raised*
- collapse
- pleurisy ±
  infarction
- ascites
- postoperative
Screening necessary

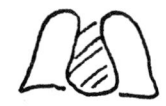

(b) *Low and 'flat'*
- hyperinflation

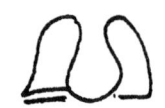

(c) *'Gas' underneath*
- ruptured viscus
- subdiaphragmatic abscess

Abnormalities produced by abdominal organs

Liver:

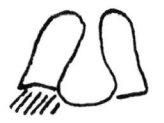

Raises diaphragm especially when
- ascites
- abscess

Spleen:

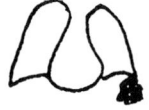

Visualized normally in up to 20% film if clinically palpated, then significant

Upper GI tract disorders:

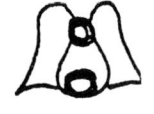

Upper
enlargement mediastinum, e.g. in pouch
Lower
Shadow behind heart, e.g. in hiatus hernia

4

Catarrhal children

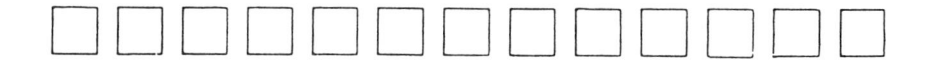

☐ ☐ ☐ ☐ ☐ ☐ ☐ ☐ ☐ ☐ ☐ ☐

SIGNIFICANCE

- Important syndrome in general because of its frequency, persistence and incomplete response to therapy.
- Risk of permanent damage.
- The term 'catarrh' is frequently used by the public. However, it may be near the truth, representing overreaction of respiratory mucosa to environmental irritants.
- There is probably no special physical make-up which predisposes the child to these special types of reactions, but rather non-specific immunological responses.

WHAT IS IT?

- Characteristic age prevalence:
    peak at 4–8 years;
    natural remission after age 8 years.
    nasal catarrh 0.5% for all ages;
    chronic bronchitis 0.2% for all ages.

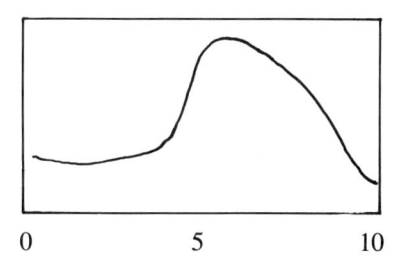

- Probably infections but specific pathogens isolated only from a proportion: 25–50%.

A catarrhal child

- Sex
- Seropurulent discharge
- Cough
- Ill-looking
- ? Seasonal variation

- Boys = girls
- Often chronic
- 'Loose' and productive
- Poor appetite, pale, failure to thrive
- Slightly more common in winter

PROBLEMS

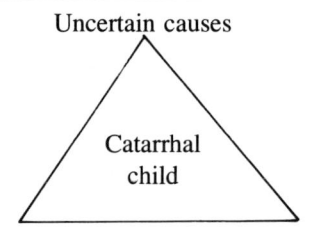

Uncertain causes

△ Catarrhal child

Difficulty in precise diagnosis   Uncertain treatment

Clinical types

- Coughs and colds (URI)
- Croup
- Acute wheezy chests
- Sore throats
- Earache ± discharge

TREATMENT

General plan

- Assessment of the condition to decide on treatment, i.e.
  (1) degree of illness,
  (2) special signs.
- Choice
  (1) Explain to parents
  (2) Relief of symptoms

(3) Specific
  - antibiotics
  - surgery
(4) Importance of follow-up.

Assessment (General)	
• Clinical examination and history	• Include ENT and swabs for bacteriology Immunological tests in a few
• Chest X-ray	• If there is doubt in diagnosis, or other serious chest conditions suspected
• Allergy tests	• Useful when family history of allergy
• Social factors	• Help from school medical officer, nurse and parents

Specific choice

- Bacteria colonizing catarrhal lesions are not primary causes of catarrhal conditions. In some children, elimination of mixed secondary bacterial invasion would be logical and *surgical treatment* will bring satisfactory results. Irreversible tissue damage is observed with specimens of tonsils, adenoids etc removed in those 'judged suitable for surgical treatment'.

- Most upper respiratory tract infections are mild, short-lived and uncomplicated, therefore antibiotics, vitamins and 'tonics' not necessary.

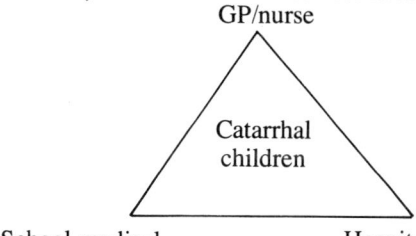

```
                    GP/nurse
                       /\
                      /  \
                     / Catarrhal \
                    /  children   \
                   /_____\
   School medical                Hospital physician/health visitor
   officer                       ± ENT surgeon
```

- The general practitioner at most advantage – has intimate knowledge of family relationships and circumstances.

- Parents' emotional reactions may lead to unnecessary investigations and treatment. Children may react to 'overprotection' by exaggerating symptoms to avoid school; therefore support the parents by explanation and reassurance. Sympathy needed.

- Avoid overclothing, coddling and overheating the homes – education and dietary advice important.

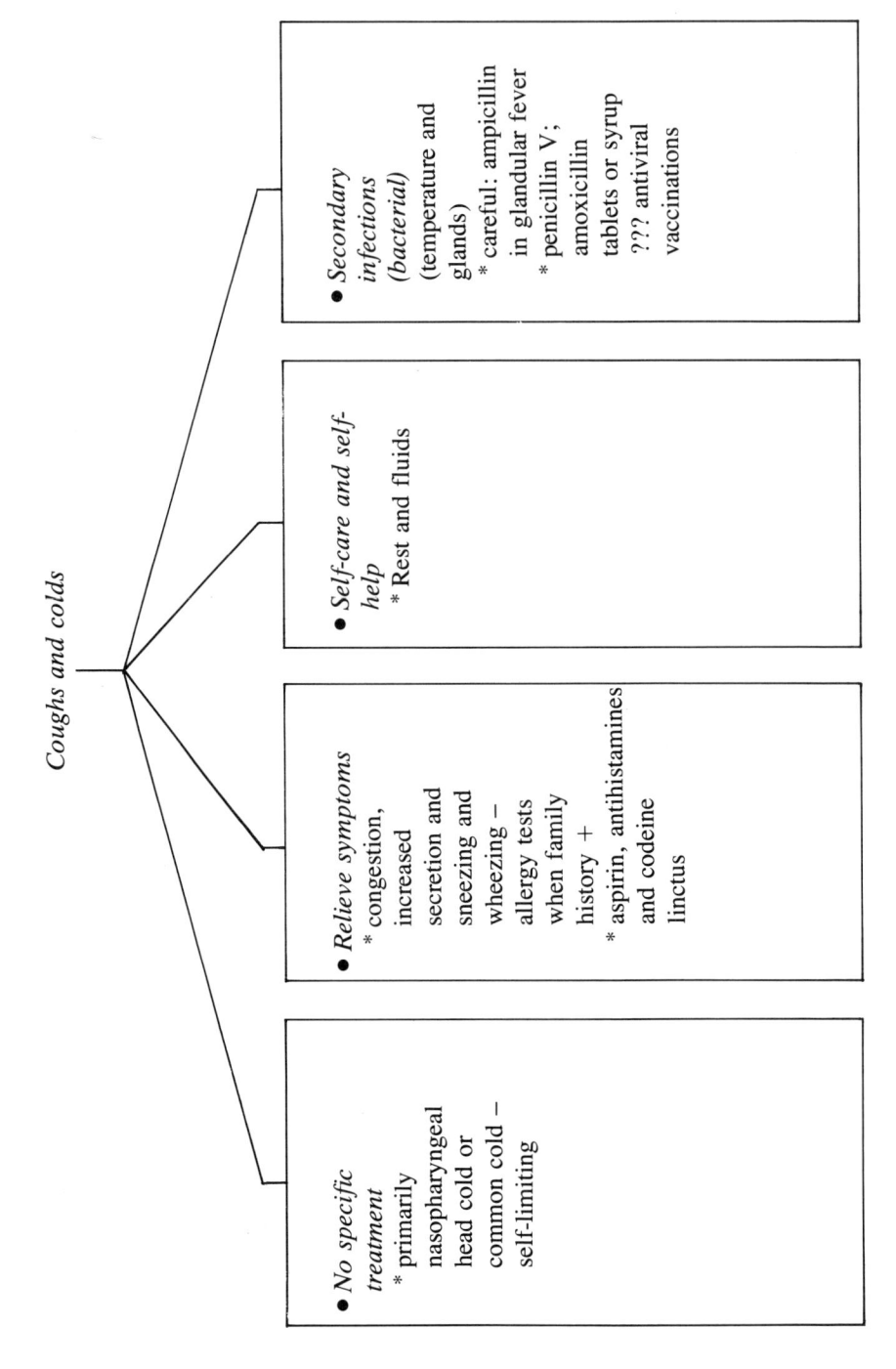

RESPIRATORY DISEASES

Coughs and colds

- **No specific treatment**
  * primarily nasopharyngeal head cold or common cold – self-limiting

- **Relieve symptoms**
  * congestion, increased secretion and sneezing and wheezing – allergy tests when family history +
  * aspirin, antihistamines and codeine linctus

- **Self-care and self-help**
  * Rest and fluids

- **Secondary infections (bacterial)** (temperature and glands)
  * careful: ampicillin in glandular fever
  * penicillin V; amoxicillin tablets or syrup
  ??? antiviral vaccinations

CROUP

- No specific therapy
- Relief of symptoms
- Reassure and explain to parents
- Risks of acute laryngeal obstruction (less than 5%)
- Differential diagnosis: epiglottitis

Acute wheezy chests

Features
- Wheezing a common accompaniment of bronchitis – estimated 25% constitutional upset with fever

- Not a forerunner of asthma

- Causes
  ? bacterial
  ? viral
  ? hypersensitivity

Management
- Explain significance to parents. Bronchodilators: short courses
  * salbutamol (tablets & syrup)
  * theophylline (tablets & syrup)
  * pressurized inhalers not necessary
  * antihistamines at night
  * steroids very rarely

- A few cases associated with fibrocystic disease, immunoglobulin deficiency and congenital heart disease

- Antibiotics: bacterial infections
  * penicillin
  * amoxicillin
  * ampicillin
  Careful follow-up

Sore throats

Features
- Frequent symptom in a catarrhal child

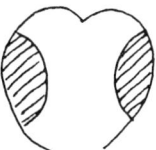

- Appearance unrelated to causes:
  viral
  bacterial
  immune-deficiency

Management
- Explain; antibiotics when constitutional symptoms and evidence of infection.
  * penicillin oral/parenteral
  * ampicillin oral
  * amoxicillin oral

- Tonsillectomy in recurrent symptoms with morbidity

> *A catarrhal child: summary*
>
> (1) Acute (common cold) and chronic (nasal discharge and cough) is *predominantly a winter condition* – sharp rise in September – *when children return to school*
>
> (2) *Infants and small children* more likely to be *susceptible*
>
> (3) ?? Social factors
>
> (4) ? Individual susceptibility – allergic diathesis
>
> (5) Management has to be pragmatic but sensible – *not all caused by antibiotic sensitive pathogens*

5

Chronic bronchitis and emphysema

☐ ☐ ☐ ☐ ☐ ☐ ☐ ☐ ☐ ☐ ☐ ☐

AIRWAYS OBSTRUCTION AND REVERSIBILITY

Significance

Chronic airways obstruction results from several disorders – so-called chronic obstructive airways disease (COAD)

(1) Bronchial asthma } potentially reversible
(2) Wheezy bronchitis } (*see* Chapter 6, Bronchial Asthma)

(3) Chronic bronchitis }
(4) Emphysema } potentially irreversible
(5) Bronchiectasis }

(For Bronchiectasis *see* Chapter 12, Chronic Infections of the Lungs.)

- *Chronic bronchitis* is defined as a disease in which there is a cough and sputum for 2–3 months in a year (usually during winter) for at least 2 consecutive years – in absence of any other recognizable conditions.
- *Emphysema* is strictly a clinicopathological diagnosis characterized by large, broken-down air sacs and terminal bronchioles – resulting in abnormal exchange of oxygen and carbon dioxide.

- *Mortality* trends over the last 10 years in 55–64 age group with COAD: highest risk during winter months:

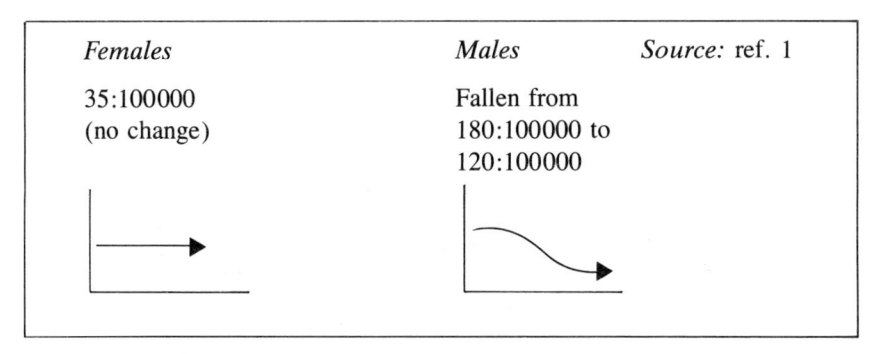

Females	*Males*	*Source:* ref. 1
35:100000 (no change)	Fallen from 180:100000 to 120:100000	

- There is steady increase in mortality with increasing urbanization. However, control of atmospheric pollution, especially in London, over the last 15 years has resulted in a fall in death rates amongst males (50–59 y).

Causal factors
- Cigarette consumption
- Occupation
- Inheritance
- Infections
- Pollution

The effects of 'smoke' inhaled either as a result of cigarette consumption or atmospheric pollution are the same – increased mucus production and retention causing cough and sputum. Therefore smokers in polluted environment run increased risk. Parents who smoke may predispose their children to infections and these individuals are susceptible to so called 'wheezy bronchitis' in later years even if they remain non-smokers.

CHRONIC BRONCHITIS AND EMPHYSEMA

What are they?

NORMAL

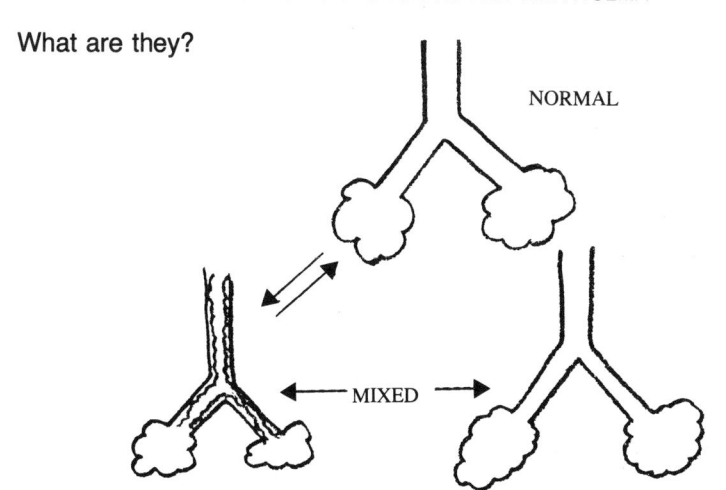

◄— MIXED —►

Chronic bronchitis

Pathology
  large and small airways
  hyperplasia of mucus
  oedema/fibrosis
  exudate – mucoid

Emphysema

Centriacinar (centrilobular)
  distended respiratory
  bronchioles
Panacinar (panlobular)
  all airways and alveoli
  involved

Clinical features

Chronic bronchitis and emphysema	
Symptoms	*Signs*
• *Cough and sputum* Patient may have been doing so for years but will usually present blaming a 'recent' infection. Haemoptysis very rare	• In early stages there may be *no signs*
	• Acute exacerbation may reveal *fever* and *crackles* at lung bases (end-inspiratory)
• *Wheeze and dyspnoea* This will invariably follow in later stages especially of emphysema	• *Clubbing* unusual
	• Chest *hyperinflated* and *hyperresonant*
• *Tiredness, lethargy and decrease in exercise tolerance* In severe cases characterized by significant hypoxia or heart failure. These symptoms usually result in 'time off work'	• May be *pursing the lips* and using *accessory muscles of respiration*
	• *Complications* of respiratory and cardiac failure (*cor pulmonale*) – see below

Investigations

- *History* and *examination*, as stated, most important.
- *Chest X-ray* is often normal.
  In some:

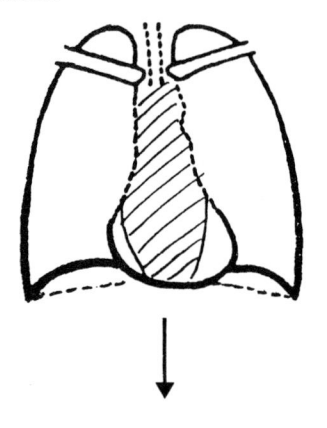

Hyperinflation with narrow heart

Increase basal or apical lucency (α_1-antitrypsin deficiency)

Unilateral hyperlucency with small pulmonary vessels (Macleod's syndrome)

Flattened diaphragms

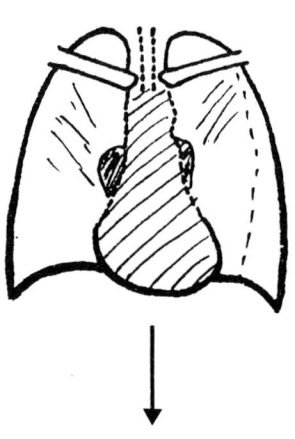

Increase in the size of heart with prominence of hilar vasculature − cor pulmonale

Pneumothorax (a small collapse can cause devastating effect in chronic severe cases)

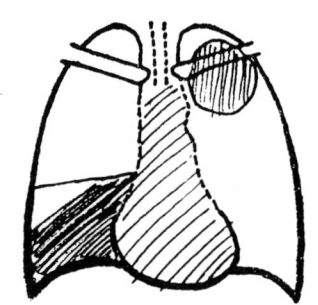

Complications of pneumonia, TB, cancer, rib fracture (coughing, steroids)

Large/small bullae or cysts (congenital)

CHRONIC BRONCHITIS AND EMPHYSEMA

- *Sputum examination*
  (1) In *recurrent infections*; culture may help choice of therapy (drug)
  (2) *Exclusion of other respiratory disorders* e.g. asthma, tumour, TB, unusual infection – e.g. mycobacterium (anonymous) and aspergillus
- *Lung function tests*: PEFR, FEV_1, FVC
  (1) To assess reversibility
  (2) To monitor response to therapy
- *Blood tests*: Full blood count
  High haemoglobin and PCV suggesting secondary polycythaemia. May benefit from venesection. High eosinophil count – to exclude allergy syndrome
- *Electrocardiograph*
  (1) Low voltage record is very common due to hyperinflated chest
  (2) May indicate right ventricular hypertrophy

I	II	III	aVR	aVL	aVF

V_1	2	3	4	5	6

Problems

- The clinical presentation of chronic bronchitis and emphysema ranges in severity from a mild disability in simple chronic bronchitis, to a severe disability with chronic respiratory failure associated with either bronchitis and/or emphysema. Development of cor pulmonale (right heart failure secondary to airways obstruction) is a poor prognostic index. Leg oedema may be the first sign of this.
- Although chronic bronchitis usually coexists with emphysema, there are patients with symptoms predominant of one or the other. How to distinguish?
- Of the 20% general practitioner consultations in adults due to respiratory disorders, two thirds will be either due to acute exacerbation of chronic bronchitis and emphysema or chronic disability from them. Whom to refer for further advice and what specific questions to ask?

RESPIRATORY DISEASES

- As chronic bronchitis and emphysema are irreversible, what indications for 'bronchodilators'?
- Is there a group to benefit from oral or parenteral steroids?
- Oxygen therapy – who will benefit?
- Use of antibiotics – when and what?
- Prophylaxis against recurrent infective episodes – antibiotics and 'flu' vaccines.
- What 'place' for physiotherapy and 'breathing exercises'?
- Patient education – what, and who to do it?
- Surgical treatment – choice of patients. For what treatment?
- Mucolytic agents – what help in treatment?
- Tobacco produces and aggravates chronic bronchitis and emphysema – yet there is no evidence that total consumption is decreasing.

Predominance of chronic bronchitis

- Definite *previous history of cough and sputum* for many years. By the time they present, cough is continuous.
- *Heavy cigarette* consumption.
- Often *overweight, cyanosed* ('the blue bloater').
- *No apparent distress at rest*; respiratory rate is normal or very slightly increased. High/normal Hb (secondary polycythaemia).
- *Slightly hyperinflated* chest which on auscultation reveals *polyphonic wheezes* and *end-inspiratory crackles* which may *disappear on coughing*.
- Evidence of *right heart failure* in late stages.
- Reduced PEFR (usually less than 200 l/min). *Minute volume* and *transfer factor* are normal.
- 'Blue bloaters' show
  low $P_{O_2} \approx 8$ kPa
  normal or high $P_{CO_2} \approx 6-8$ kPa

Predominance of emphysema

- Long history of *exertional dyspnoea* and *reduction in exercise tolerance* – may be confused with cardiac disorders. *Cough is minimal* – very little sputum.
- Usually moderate-to-heavy cigarette consumer. Note α_1-antitrypsin deficiency (*see below*).
- Often *asthenic, puffing* (tachypnoea), *pursed lips,* leaning forward with arms stretched to brace himself – *'Pink puffer'* – *distressed at rest*.

CHRONIC BRONCHITIS AND EMPHYSEMA

- Neck veins may dilate on expiration only. Very hyperinflated chest, *hyperresonance especially at bases*. Very few polyphonic wheezes. *Heart sounds faint* with a gallop rhythm.
- Total lung capacity and residual volume increased. *Transfer factor decreased*. PEFR very low < 120 l/min. Impaired elastic recoil.
- 'Pink puffers' show
  low $P_{O_2} \approx$ 6–8 kPa
  low $P_{CO_2} \approx$ 4 kPa

α_1-Antitrypsin deficient emphysema

- *What patient?*

- *Measurement?*
  Most people have levels in excess of 250 mg/100 ml (genotype *MM*)

- *When relevant?*
  (in emphysema two genes *Z* and *S*)

- Family screening

- Treatment
  (get advice from specialist)

- Young, male, ? smoker with family history. Chest X-ray: basal hyperlucency ± bullae

- An ordinary clotted 10 ml of blood required

- Homozygous *ZZ* or *SS*
  < 50 mg/100 ml panacinar emphysema ♂ = ♀ heterozygotes *MZ* or *MS* 50–100 mg/100 ml (may or may not develop emphysema)

- In severe cases – screening would reveal those with low levels – (1) assess yearly, (2) stop them smoking

- Steroids useful. *Do* detailed lung function tests (inc. transfer factor) and monitor progress 6-monthly

MANAGEMENT OF ACUTE EPISODES

Patients with chronic irreversible airways obstruction will be prone to more and more acute exacerbations as the disease progresses. These may range from *mild* increase in the common symptoms of cough, sputum and dyspnoea – easily dealt with by the patient at home – to *moderate* disability when a general practitioner will be consulted. When *severe* and *prostrating* illness ensues – e.g. pneumonia, pneumothorax or heart failure – the patient will be referred to hospital for assessment, especially regarding oxygen therapy. Excess oxygen supplement – without facilities for blood gases analysis and assisted ventilation – could be very hazardous and wasteful.

Infections

In the majority, exacerbations will follow cold, 'flu' or other viral illness during the time when there is increased atmospheric pollution (winter months).

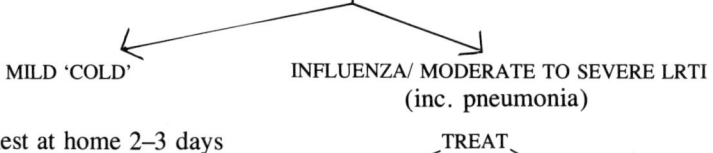

MILD 'COLD' →
INFLUENZA/ MODERATE TO SEVERE LRTI (inc. pneumonia)

- Rest at home 2–3 days
- Hydration, nutrition

TREAT → AT HOME / IN HOSPITAL

Increase in sputum (purulent) with constitutional symptoms
Give ampicilillin 250 mg q.d.s for 7 days

or

Co-trimoxazole 2 b.d. for 7 days

Trimethoprim alone is equally useful.

For *bronchodilators: see below.*

Do not give 'cough' mixtures containing antihistamines and

AT HOME:
- Uncomplicated
- Previously well
- Give ampicillin or amoxicillin 250 mg q.d.s 7 days

bronchodilators
oxygen
hydrate

IN HOSPITAL:
- Complicated
- Oxygen dependent
- Those failing to respond at home after 48 h

sedatives ⟶ most cause drowsiness and retention of sputum

Choice of antibiotic for acute exacerbation

- *Common bacteria* responsible for attacks:

    Haemophilus influenzae ⎫
    Streptococcus pneumoniae ⎬ may occur together

- *Uncommon organisms*

    Klebsiella pneumoniae
    Staphylococcus
    Pseudomonas

- Sputum bacteriology *not* necessary and often confusing.
- Benzylpenicillin, streptomycin and chloramphenicol are most effective but *not* first line of drug management. These compounds are often used in hospital when home management has 'failed'. *Pseudomonas* may occur in debilitated patients and will need gentamicin and carbenicillin. Aerosol inhalation of gentamicin is useful in these.
- *Ampicillin* is effective. Do not use if glandular fever coexisting or suspected.
- *Amoxicillin* has no advantage over ampicillin and is costly – it is slightly less effective against. *H. influenzae*.
- *Tetracycline* and *erythromycin*, although slightly inferior than ampicillin, may be useful in 'atypical pneumonias'. There are tetracycline-resistant strains of *H. influenzae*, and erythromycin may produce jaundice.
- *Chloramphenicol* used as 250–500 mg four times a day can be effective in some, and should be tried when patients' comfort outweighs risks of pancytopenia. Regular (every second day) FBC and white cell count is necessary.
- *Co-trimoxazole* not favoured, as resistant *H. influenzae* strains have been identified.

WHAT USE ARE BRONCHODILATORS?

- Bronchospasm will be particularly evident in acute exacerbation.
- It is useful to assess reversibility in the early stages by undertaking measurement of PEFR and Vitalograph (if available) – the patient is then given a measured dose of bronchodilator (200 μg (two puffs) of salbutamol or 0.16 mg isoprenaline) and the tests repeated at 5, 20 minutes. If improvement is over 20%, suspect asthma.

  Many patients with chronic bronchitis and emphysema reverse between 5 and 10%. These will be suitable for either long-term or short-term bronchodilator therapy.
- Give a small dose initially as side-effects common.

Drugs (bronchodilators) used

Acute episode

When *very wheezy* give i.v. 200–500 mg *aminophylline* slowly preferably monitoring pulse (10–15 min). Give oxygen concurrently if possible. Repeat 6–8 hourly if necessary. *Do not* use i.m. preparations (less effective and painful).

Inhalation (via *nebulizer* or IPPB) 2.5 ml of *salbutamol*. Repeat 6–8 hourly until patient better. *Do not* give i.v. salbutamol (induces complex biochemical reactions).

Chronic disease

SR aminophylline 225–450 mg twice a day (well tolerated at small doses). Useful in early morning symptoms. Proprietary preparations: Uniphyllin, Slo-phyllin, Nuelin, Theo-odor.

Salbutamol and terbutaline tabs, syrup and inhalation.

Steroid inhalers should not be used.

Atropine derivatives; ipratropium inhaler may improve airflow.

ORAL AND PARENTERAL STEROIDS

- May be useful in *young patients* with α_1-*antitrypsin* deficiency emphysema. If no improvement after 3 months (judge on 'detail' lung function tests) – *stop*.

- When the diagnosis is in doubt or where there is well substantiated reversibility of 10–15%, trial of steroids may be useful and may result in dramatic effect.

- In most chronic bronchitics and emphysema patients, corticosteroids are unhelpful and may cause problems in future with adrenal suppression, immunosuppression (infections with unusual organisms), reactivation of tuberculosis and Cushing's syndrome. Oral and laryngeal and lower respiratory tract *Candida* increase the problems as the patient may also receive frequent courses of antibiotics.

What steroid?

If possible add steroid to the treatment regime without altering the schedule – to see objective improvement (measure PEFR and FEV_1 daily)

Oral, give

    prednisone 30 mg daily for 1st week
    prednisone 20 mg daily for 2nd week
    prednisone 10 mg daily for 2 weeks

Assess. If improvement, continue 5 mg/day for 6–12 weeks, then gradually withdraw and give during exacerbation.

Parenteral, give

triamcinolone 80 mg i.m.

Repeat every 4 weeks for 3 months

Assess. If improvement, continue at 6-weekly intervals for further 3 months – then withdraw except in 'severe' cases where quality of life is significantly better on 'them'.

Hydrocortisone 100–200 mg 8-hourly in exacerbation only.

Depomedrone; ACTH *should not* be used.
ACTH causes adrenal suppression
Depomedrone *not* effective

OXYGEN

- It is undoubtedly *indicated in acute exacerbation* of chronic bronchitis and emphysema. It is of special benefit when used with intravenous aminophylline and nebulized salbutamol. However, patients retaining CO_2 may progress further into respiratory failure if the amount used is *not* monitored. Therefore importance of regular blood gas measurement. If not, use 24–28% via Venti- or Edinburgh mask.
- Do *not* prescribe sedatives, especially *morphia*, as patients with chronic hypercapnia depend on the hypoxic drive to continue to 'respire'.
- Oxygen in many patients will increase the exercise tolerance and improve the quality of life on long term.

Long-term use of oxygen

(1) *Ordinary cylinder:*
- a domiciliary device for daily use
- heavy and cumbersome
- frequent replacement necessary
- 'pressure' not enough to nebulize, therefore a special multiflow regulator necessary (*NOT PRESCRIBED ON NHS*), available from BOC or De-Vilbiss, London approx. £70

(2) *'Portable' cylinder:*
- Small, easy to carry ($2\frac{1}{2}$ lb)
- Strapped to the back, mounted on Zimmer frame
- Frequent refilling
- Costly (rarely prescribed on NHS); obtained from BOC or De-Vilbiss, London.

(3) *Oxygen concentrator* (from room air):
- Safe, effective device, 'infant' stage of use.
- Very costly.

ANTIBIOTIC IN PROPHYLAXIS

- Drug used
ampicillin:	1 g/day divided doses
tetracycline:	1 g/day divided doses
Kelfizine-W:	2 g/week.
- Significant reduction in episodes of acute bronchitis but no evidence that it reduces the deterioration of pulmonary function [2] [3].
- Long-term co-trimoxazole (Septrin) produces drug resistant *H. influenzae*.
- Prophylaxis is expensive and should only be used in patients with significant bronchiectasis as well.
- Easier to supply the patient with antibiotics and encourage to take 'early' in an event of infective exacerbation.
- Flu vaccine should be used in 'susceptible' individuals.

PHYSIOTHERAPY; PATIENT EDUCATION; POSTURE

- Controversial but *'placebo effect'* undoubted.
- May *calm* and *give confidence* in the ability to control his/her symptoms.
- *Exercise training* with *oxygen* of value in some.
- *Postural* drainage when *sputum expectoration* is a problem.
- *Expectorants* and *mucolytic agents* – in the majority *as good* as exercises and physiotherapy.
- Chronic bronchitis and emphysema more often affect the unskilled who will eventually be unable to work. Early help (through a social worker) is invaluable. Advice will be sought regarding alteration in job environment and housing. (*See* Neilson and Crofton (1965). *The Social Aspects of Chronic Bronchitis*. (London: The Chest and Heart Association).)

SURGICAL TREATMENT

- A large emphysematous bulla (space greater than 1 cm) may be removed surgically with some improvement in lung function. These patients should be referred either to a chest physician or a surgeon.
- Small bullae usually cause pneumothorax.

- Lung scans will suggest bullae and show differential lung function as a result of these.
- A giant bulla or cyst in an infant may cause severe dyspnoea and surgical removal mandatory.

MUCOLYTIC AGENTS

Mucolytic agents are widely used in chronic bronchitis. They are expensive.

   Do they benefit the patient?
   Should the use be encouraged?
   To answer the above questions, consider

The pathology of airways
Chronic bronchitis and emphysema

• *Exudate*	• Mainly mucus
• *Mucosa/submucosa*	• Mild metaplasia
	• Increased goblet cells
• *Basement membrane*	• Somewhat thickened
• *Muscle*	• Usually normal

Mucolytic agents are thought to reduce the viscosity and elasticity of mucus – thus facilitating expectoration and reducing airway resistance.

   Assess effect of treatment:

(1) changes in symptoms
(2) improvement in lung function tests.

What agents?

Alevaire (Tyloxapol) inhalation

- Withdrawn by the US Food and Drug Administration – insufficient evidence of its usefulness. The UK Committee on Safety of Medicines yet to act.

Acetylcysteine (Airbron) inhalation

- In chronic bronchitis, shown to make mucus less viscous but may cause *bronchoconstriction in asthma* as it cleaves disulphide bonds which link glycoprotein molecules (*not recommended for wider use*).

Oral preparations

- Bromhexine tablets or elixir 8 mg b.d. or t.i.d.
- Acetylcysteine sachet 1 b.d. or at night only. *Expensive.*
- Carbocysteine syrup/capsules 750 mg t.i.d. or q.d.s. *Expensive.*

- Useful in chronic bronchitis and asthma.
- Useful in selected patients – especially in chronic bronchitis. Helps cough and dyspnoea.
- Affects mucus synthesis. No advantage over bromhexine or acetylcysteine.

SUMMARY (MUCOLYTIC AGENTS)

Further work necessary in patient selection – those who may benefit from these expensive agents.

References
1. WHO World Health Statistics Annual. (Geneva: WHO)
2. M.R.C. (1966). *Br. Med. J.*, **1,** 1317
3. Tager, I.B. *et al.* (1975). *N. Engl. J. Med.*, **292,** 563

6

Bronchial asthma

☐ ☐ ☐ ☐ ☐ ☐ ☐ ☐ ☐ ☐ ☐ ☐

SIGNIFICANCE

- Asthma is thought to occur in 5–10% of the population.[1]
- Estimated 2 million asthmatics in the UK, 6–8 million in the USA.
- Approximately 1200 deaths each year due to asthma in the UK, 6000 deaths in the USA.
- Greatest danger of death during an acute severe attack.
- Asthma is an unpredictable disorder – in the sort of person it affects, in its clinical course, response to treatment and prognosis.
- Many *children* with asthma can expect spontaneous remission of symptoms by the time of puberty. Asthma developing in *adult* life will respond to individualized treatment in a large proportion. Chronic severe asthma is a disabling condition carrying a high morbidity and mortality.
- Many asthmatics will give a previous history of wheezy bronchitis (especially in childhood) or will admit to hay fever, eczema and asthma in members of the family.
- Many significant differences in asthma as it presents in childhood and affecting adults (*see below*).
- Main types are
    (1) extrinsic (atopic)
    (2) intrinsic (non-atopic)
    (3) exercise induced
    (4) occupational
    (5) associated with other medical disorders

Extrinsic (atopic) asthma[2]

- Age — Usually a child or teenager
- Previous history — Of eczema and hay fever, either in the child or in the family
- ? Antigenic stimulus — May be found to have specific allergic response to dust, dust-mite, pollen, grass, drugs or foods
- Allergy (skin tests) — Usually positive (may respond to hyposensitization)
- Immunoglobulins — IgE associated
- Management — Mast-cell stabilizers useful, e.g. disodium cromoglycate, beclomethasone inhaler
- Prognosis — Acute attacks followed by a relatively symptom-free period. Overall prognosis favourable

Extrinsic asthma

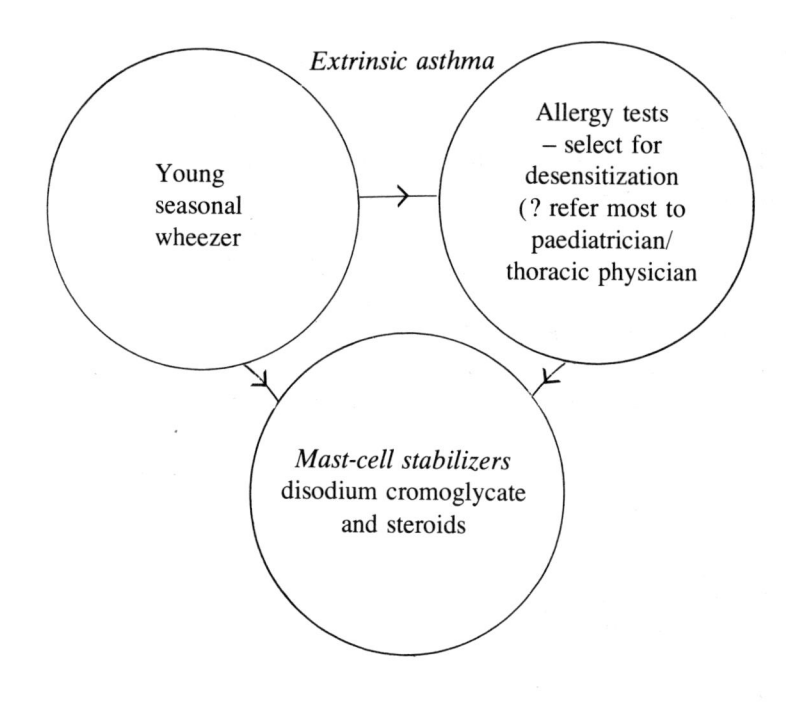

- Young seasonal wheezer
- Allergy tests — select for desensitization (? refer most to paediatrician/thoracic physician)
- *Mast-cell stabilizers* disodium cromoglycate and steroids

Intrinsic (non-atopic) asthma

- Age — Usually an adult
- Previous history — Often negative except for nasal polyps
- ? Antigen stimulus — Negative in most; some show reaction (significant) to house dust and house dust-mite
- Allergy (skin tests) — Negative (unfavourable response to hyposensitization)
- Immunoglobulins — IgE normal
- Management — Mast-cell stabilizers of no benefit
- Prognosis — Variable. Attacks often frequent. Death may occur

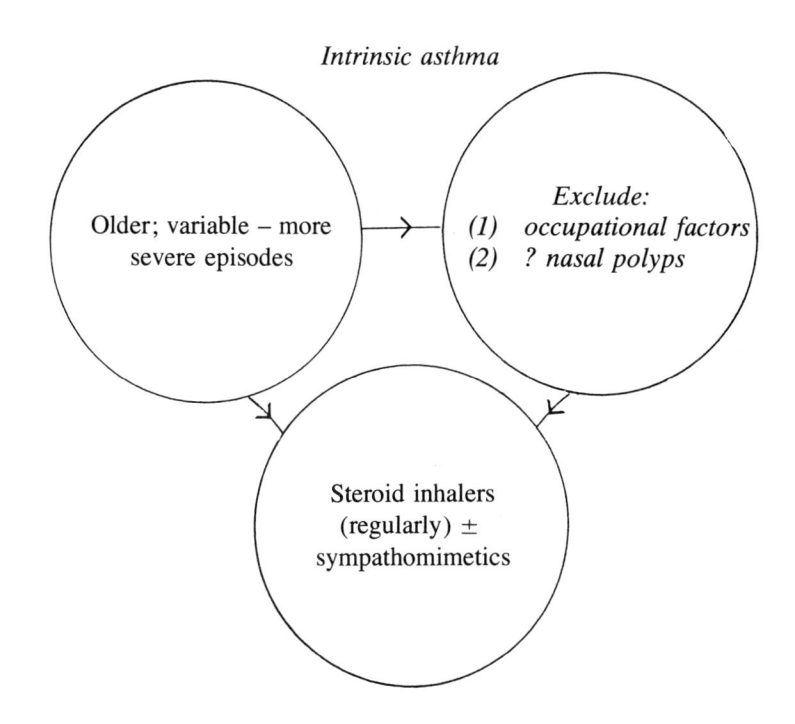

Intrinsic asthma

- Older; variable – more severe episodes
- Exclude:
  (1) *occupational factors*
  (2) *? nasal polyps*
- Steroid inhalers (regularly) ± sympathomimetics

Exercise-induced asthma

- Age
- Previous history
- ? Antigen stimulus

- Allergy and skin tests

- Immunoglobulins
- Management

- Prognosis

- Any age; commoner in children
- Patient may give history of atopy
- Precise mechanisms not defined. May be as a result of 'cold air'
- Will vary – whether the patient atopic or non-atopic
- IgE ↑↓ or normal
- Inhalation of β_2-agonist before exercise helpful
- Good

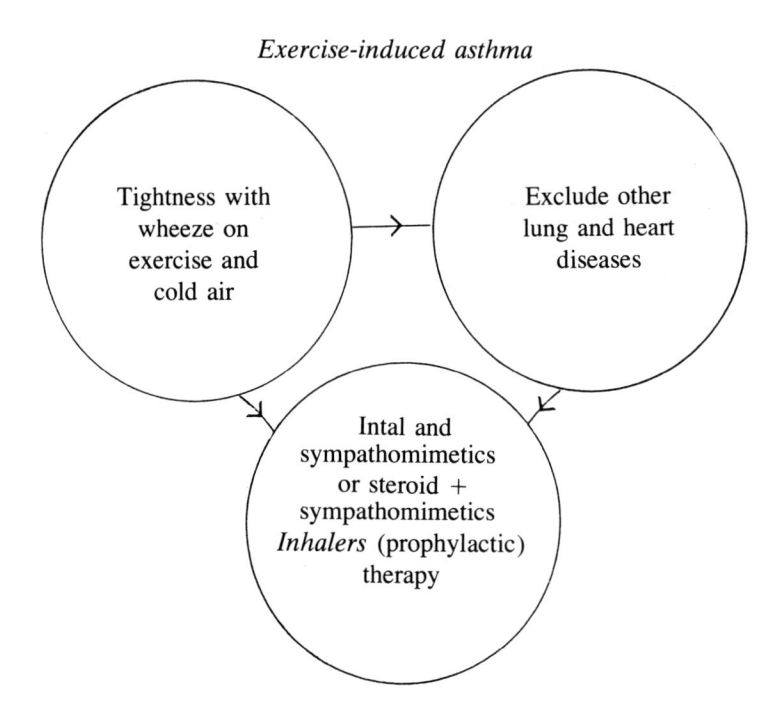

Exercise-induced asthma

- Tightness with wheeze on exercise and cold air
- Exclude other lung and heart diseases
- Intal and sympathomimetics or steroid + sympathomimetics *Inhalers* (prophylactic) therapy

Occupational asthma

Type	Agent
• Detergent trade	• *Bacillus subtilis*
• Carpenters	• Wood dusts
• Printing	• Vegetable gums
• Coffee workers	• Coffee bean
• Textile industry	• Cotton dust
• Bakers	• Grain and flour
• Pharmaceutical industry	• Penicillin, cimetidine, piperazine, sulphonamides
• Veterinary/bird fanciers	• Sera and secretions
• Chemicals (industrials)	• Isocyanates, solders, dyes, persulphates
• Metal refining	• Platinum, nickel, chromium

Occupational asthma

Wheezing on the job. Do not forget the spouse → Most at risk: Farmers, bakers, pharmaceutical industry, housewife (detergents)

↓ ↓

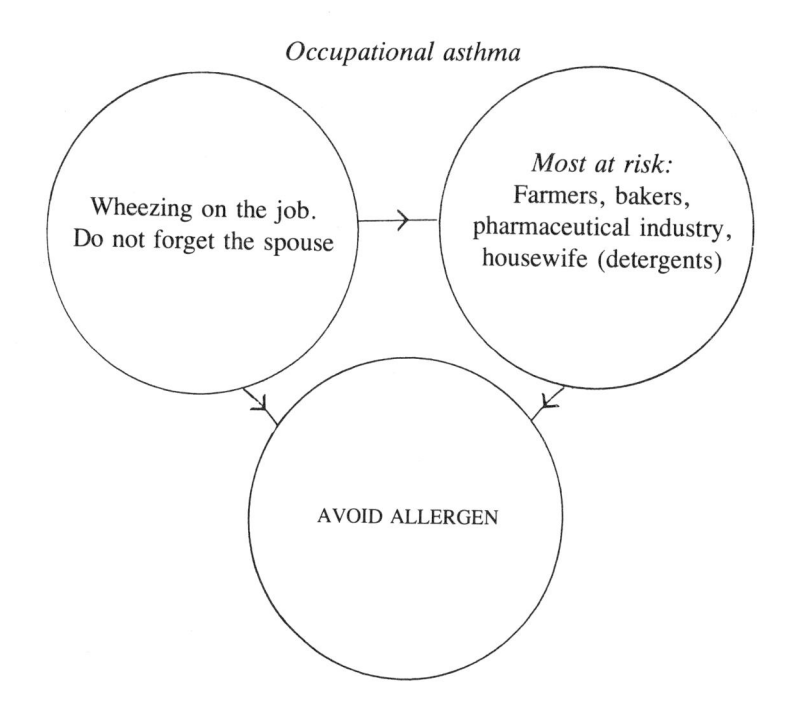

AVOID ALLERGEN

Asthma associated with other disorders

Type	Features
• Chronic pulmonary aspergillosis	• Respiratory disability due to *Aspergillus fumigatus*: pneumonia (recurrent) steroids necessary
• Polyarteritis nodosa	• Systemic condition. Very high ESR and eosinophilic count.
• Eosinophilic granuloma	• Commoner in children: premalignant recurrent pneumonia

The pathology of airways
Bronchial asthma

• Exudate	• Eosinophils (asthma stigmata)
• Mucosa/submucosa	• Metaplasia (prominent)
	• Oedema/vasodilatation
• Basement membrane	• Greatly thickened
• Muscle	• Hypertrophy

ASTHMA IN CHILDREN

1. Epidemiology

• Common: ♂ : ♀ = 2:1	• Affects approximately 5–10% of children. If those with 'acute wheezy chests' are included, then incidence may rise to approximately 25%, i.e. 2–5 times that in young adults[3]. Over two thirds of children with asthma will have symptoms by the age of 5 years.
• Progress	• 25% episodic symptoms / 33% get better / 2.5% severe / ?
• Mortality	• Low (45 deaths/annum)

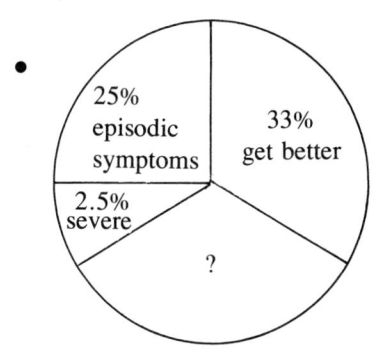

2. Types [4]

Acute wheezy bronchitis	Bronchial asthma
• Cough and wheeze following 'viral' infections. RSV isolated in some	• Cough and wheeze (seasonal, at night and on exercise)
• Hypoxia – rare	• Life-threatening hypoxia may occur
• Course < 5 days	• Course > 5 days
• Usually stop after 14 years	• Prognosis unpredictable

• Management: supportive:
   Hydrate
   Closely observe
   Steroids not necessary
   Antibiotics in very few
	• Treatment with bronchodilators effective

3. Management of childhood asthma

• Try to identify stimulus	• Good history is more important
	• Allergic (patch testing in selected cases)
	• Emotional ? hypnosis
	• Physical, e.g. exercise
	• Infective
• Lung function tests	• Measure PEFR several times a day and assess reversibility
• Exclude other disorder	• Sweat test (cystic fibrosis)
	• Eosinophil count (blood) (pulmonary eosinophilia and eosinophilic granuloma)
• Lifestyle	• Normal school and activity in most
	• Avoid proven allergens
• Drugs	• As in adults (*see below*)

ASTHMA IN ADULTS

1. Epidemiology

• Common: ♀ : ♂ = 2:1	• Affects approximately 7–10%
• Progress	• Variable/unpredictable especially in intrinsic asthma
• Mortality	• Significant (1200 deaths/annum)

2. Types

Wheezy bronchitis	Bronchial asthma
• Cough, wheeze and sputum usually in winter following URTI	• Cough, wheeze, 'glue'-like sputum (very little)
• Usually a smoker	• Often a non-smoker
• Partially reversible airflow obstruction	• Reversible airflow obstruction
• Hypoxia and high P_{CO_2} may occur	• Blood gases abnormal in 'severe' episodes
• Acute episode $\approx$ 10/14 days	• Unpredictable course
• Heart failure may occur	• Heart failure: rare
• Bronchodilators and steroids in moderate/severe cases. Not always helpful. Antibiotics necessary	• Bronchodilators – effective

3. Management of adult asthma

• Try to identify stimulus	• Relevant mostly in occupational asthma
• Lung function tests	• Measure PEFR. Demonstrate variability. Low value in early morning – 'dip'
• Exclude other disorders	• Neoplasm
	• Polyarteritis nodosa (high ESR, eosinophil count) and renal involvement
	• Aspergillosis (skin tests, precipitins)
• Lifestyle	• Most can lead a normal life
• Drugs	• *See below*

CLINICAL FEATURES

- Defined as a condition characterized by paroxysmal wheezing with dyspnoea, cough and viscid sputum. It is reversible with time and appropriate management. The peak expiratory flow rate *(PEFR) in litres/min rises by over 20% following 200 µg of salbutamol or 0.16 mg of isoprenaline.*
- Flushing, cyanosis, use of accessory respiratory muscles, confusion/aggression and tachycardia present especially in acute attacks.

RESPIRATORY DISEASES

- Chest X-ray often normal but may show a *pneumothorax* or *bronchopulmonary aspergillosis*.
- Some degree of *eosinophilia* (blood) found in atopic form.
  Sputa often show *stigmata of asthma:*
  Curschmann's spirals
  Charcot–Leyden crystals
  eosinophils.
- Hypercapnia (high P_{CO_2}) rare, therefore oxygen therapy useful and safe.

DIFFERENTIAL DIAGNOSIS OF ASTHMA

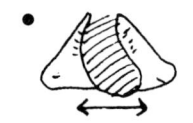

- Congestive heart failure (cardiac asthma)

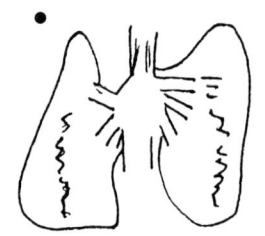

- Bronchiolitis especially in children
- Widespread granulomatous disorder, e.g. sarcoid
- Bronchiectasis
- Allergic alveolitis

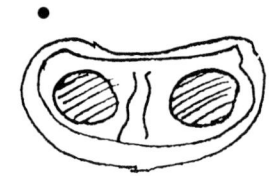

- Laryngeal oedema (croup)
- Laryngeal tumour or cyst

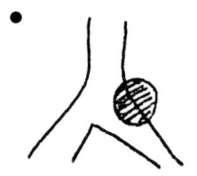

- Congenital rings
- Aneurysm/tumour
- Tracheobronchial tumours – extrinsic lymph nodes

- Pulmonary embolism
- Hiatus hernia
- Anaphylaxis
- Disproportionate dyspnoea and anxiety

> *Suspect asthma in these cases*
>
> ## ADOPT HIGH INDEX OF SUSPICION
>
> - Chronic (over 4 weeks) cough with very little viscid sputum ± wheeze
> - Symptoms particularly worse on exercise, cold air and at night
> - Tightness and wheeze developing in later life with previous history of the same or family history of eczema, asthma, hay fever
> - Wheezing, dyspnoea developing following commencement of drugs, e.g. β-blockers, aspirin
> - Wheezing and cough occurring in certain occupations, especially when person returns to work after a weekend break

> *Features rare or unusual in asthma*
>
> - Finger clubbing
> - Cyanosis (unless in very severe acute asthma, especially in elderly)
> - Respiratory failure (arterial blood gases show slightly low P_{O_2} and normal or low P_{CO_2} in most)
> - Haemoptysis (rarely after a severe bout of coughing)
> - Cor pulmonale (right heart failure secondary to chronic airways obstruction)

PROBLEMS

- Majority of asthmatics will have no definite cause; prevention not possible in most.
- Allergy influences are overemphasized. When a specific agent is identified, very little help can be offered in the programme of desensitization.
- Although occupational asthma can proceed to a serious, chronic disorder in some, patients are often reluctant to 'leave the job'.
- Uncertainty in causes often leads to 'trial and error' method of management using various inhaled, nebulized, oral and parenteral therapy available.
- Most cases of asthma should be identified and treated by general practitioners[5]. Evidence however suggests that management of asthmatics is being taken away from general practice to hospital. Between 1970 and 1978 a more than fivefold increase occurred in the number of children with acute severe asthma who were admitted to hospitals in the South-West Thames Region without the mediation of

their general practitioners[6]. Factors like difficulty in contacting 'own GP' and dislike of deputizing services, especially at night when acute attacks are likely to occur, may be responsible. Confidence in the treatment offered by GP is essential to reduce the large number of 'direct' admissions to hospital.
- Failure of the patients and at times their GPs to recognize the rapid progression of a severe attack is responsible for many asthma deaths[7].
- There is also evidence that childhood asthma is 'under-diagnosed' in general practice[8] and the management is inappropriate.
- Often when patients are referred to a specialist, they will remain in 'hospital' care – thus shifting the emphasis on management of the patient away from practice.
- The letter of referral to a specialist should cover the background history and the sort of management plans tried and failed and should ask the specialist's advice on specific uncertainties. It is also useful to state that the GP would follow the guidance and the patients should be returned back to his care.
- 'Asthma Clinics' in hospitals may be staffed by junior doctors with little experience in management and would 'change' frequently. It is very reassuring for the patient to see the same doctor as would be the case in most GP surgeries.
- Although bronchial asthma is characterized by unpredictability and there are doubts on its aetiology and best forms of treatment, a GP should be didactic and clear in the dealings with the patient.
- It is impossible to diagnose and pursue the course of bronchial asthma without measurement of a peak flow meter. Many general practices still do not possess such a basic instrument. A good control is when the patient achieves over 75% of his or her best recorded figure during a natural or induced remission.
- Emphasis in asthma should shift from prevention to appropriate treatment.

MANAGEMENT: GENERAL PRACTICE

Identify and try to eradicate allergic features.

Advise on occupational aspects – if appropriate.

Explore and treat emotional and social component.

Keep the drug therapy simple.

Improve the quality of life in the few severe chronic cases of asthma and aim for the majority to lead a normal life.

Diagnose and aim to treat acute severe asthmatics (status asthmaticus) at home if possible.

Allergic symptoms

In patients in whom allergy plays a significant role, specific hyposensitization is an important factor in long-term management. Such a programme may be inconvenient, costly, injections are painful and not always effective. Indications for hyposensitization are:

(1) when 'general avoidance' measures have failed,

(2) when drug therapy is not tolerated or is ineffective,

(3) allergy tests show very strong reaction,

(4) very high IgE levels > 150iu/ml.

Many antigens are available for testing. Some GPs have facilities to undertake these, e.g. *Bencard Diagnositc Set*. Others refer to chest clinics or dermatology departments.

Allergens to test: house dust, house dust mite, grass, pollen, aspergillus, danders and appropriate food. Measure the weal after 20 minutes. A reaction > 5 mm is regarded as positive.

Bronchial provocation tests are controversial but useful in diagnosing occupational factors. The patient will need a specialist opinion. Some patients will develop severe 'anaphylactic' symptoms during allergy testing and it would be safer to have hydrocortisone and oxygen easily available to counteract these.

House dust and mite allergy is common even in those without asthma. These patients are at their worst in the early hours of the morning. The faecal pellets of the mite lodged in the nasal passages cause secretions of substances which cause bronchospasm. Simple measures, e.g. 'hoovering', keeping the bedroom tidy and 'dusting' the sheets, may reduce the population of the mite by over 40%. *Tymasil* (natamycin) (a specific agent for the control of house dust mite) is in experimental stage. In controlled trials, up to two thirds of patients with allergy to selected pollens have been shown to improve substantially with hyposensitization. The best response is expected in young patients.

Management of allergy to animal danders is difficult. Often 'taking away' a pet from the child may cause worsening of the symptoms because of emotional stress. In these cases depot injection of methylprednisone (Depomedrone 40 mg) or triamcinolone given every 4–6 weeks, may help.

Occupational aspects

The individual should be clearly informed of the dangers.

Report (with patient's permission) to his work medical officer and employment adviser for identification of further cases.

Avoid further exposure if possible. Many will be reluctant to 'leave the job', but often sympathy from employers will be forthcoming and a change in occupation may be possible. If this fails treat the patient with drugs and closely monitor lung function tests. Hospital/GP dual care appropriate here.

Therapy is often unsuccessful and the patient may progress to severe disability and irreversible obstruction.

Emotional factors

- Hope for a 'cure' of the condition is what most patients expect. Failure to achieve this may lead to considerable anxiety. The GP should lay stress on the good prognosis and offer appropriate treatment.
- Emotional stress can precipitate an attack[9].
- Special personality or neuroticism is not shown to be very relevant in asthma.
- Emotional stress should not be blamed for failure of drug therapy.
- There are anecdotal cases when improvement has been achieved by hypnosis and physiotherapy.
- The most likely outcome is change of personality and prevention of secondary psychological disorders in appropriately treated cases.

Drug therapy

> Types
> - *Inhaled*
> - *Oral*
> - *Nebulized*
> - *Parenteral*
> - *Others*

Inhalers and spacers

- Over 11 million inhalers prescribed in UK per annum.
- Still the safest and most effective way of administration of the drug to the lungs.
- Problem in improving the amount reaching the periphery of the lung (probably no more than 20%).

BRONCHIAL ASTHMA

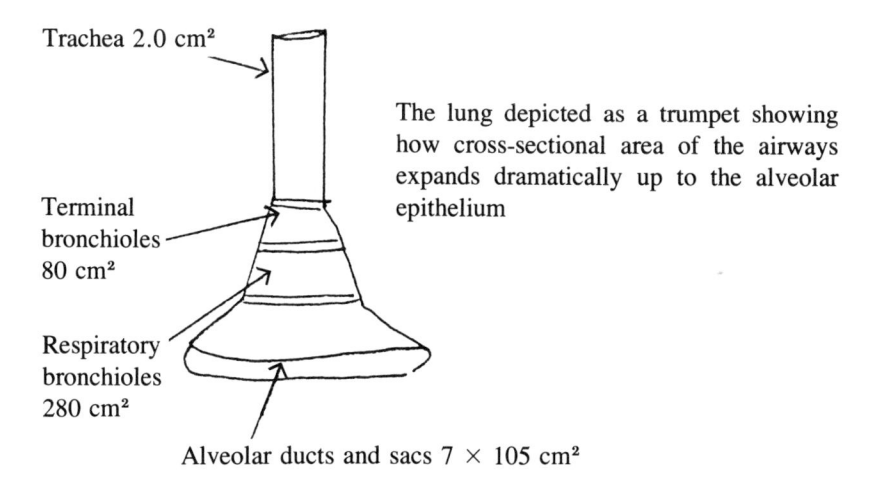

Trachea 2.0 cm²

Terminal bronchioles 80 cm²

Respiratory bronchioles 280 cm²

Alveolar ducts and sacs 7 × 105 cm²

The lung depicted as a trumpet showing how cross-sectional area of the airways expands dramatically up to the alveolar epithelium

- The elderly, the arthritic and some children will find the inhaler impossible to use. Nebulized treatment may be preferred here.
- Types are:

  β-agonist
  steroid
  anticholinergic
  combination
  sodium cromoglycate

Use of an aerosol inhaler

- Doctor should demonstrate first using a 'dummy' inhaler.
- He should watch the patient's performance and give marks between 1 and 10. Children are likely to improve on their 'score'.
- Technique:

Breathe out fully
Place the inhaler between the lips
Press the canister and inhale slowly to total lung capacity
Hold the breath for a few seconds and exhale

- A *spacer* allows the discharge of a dose to precede inspiration; a *rotahaler* is a simple breath-activated device which delivers a powdered preparation of drug. Most asthmatics do not need these. No firm evidence that delivery to the lungs increases using these types: terbutaline Spacer, salbutamol and beclamethasone.

β-Agonist inhalers

- The commonest of drugs given by inhalation[10].
- Those containing adrenaline and noradrenaline very rarely used in the UK because of their very significant 'cardiac' effects, e.g. tachyarrythmia.
- Brovon (papaverine and atropine methonitrate) inhaler still used by elderly asthmatics.
- Inhalers containing adrenaline available in USA.
- Most β-sympathomimetic inhalers help mucociliary clearance.
- Particularly useful in preventing exercise induced asthma.
- Combined with *disodium cromoglycate* will control most extrinsic childhood and adult asthma. Combined with *steroid* inhalers will control most late onset and intrinsic asthma.

Types of β_2-sympathomimetic inhalers/nebulization solution

- *Salbutamol*
  Aerosol 200 µg: 2 puffs, 4–6 times a day
  Rotacaps 200 µg 4–6 times a day
  Nebules (2.5 ml) or solution 0.1–0.5 ml in 2 ml saline, 4–6 times a day

  - Effective.
    May produce
      tachycardia
      tremor
      sweating
      headaches
      dizziness
      cramps
    Occasional idiosyncratic reaction. Avoid in thyrotoxicosis and severe ischaemic heart disease

- *Fenoterol*
  Aerosol 180 µg: (1 puff), use 2 puffs twice a day
  Nebulization solution as salbutamol but twice a day

- *Terbutaline*
  Aerosol 250–500 µg i.e. 1–2 puffs up to 4 times a day
  Nebulization solution 2–5 mg, up to 4 times a day

  - In many cases marked tremor and tachycardia

- *Rimiterol* Aerosol 200–600 µg up to 4 times a day

  - No particular advantages

- *Orciprenaline*

Types of steroid inhalers

- *Beclomethasone dipropionate* (as Becotide; Becloforte)
  Aerosol 50 μg: per puff (Becotide), 250 μg per puff (Becloforte), 2 puffs two or three times a day
  Rotacaps 100/200 μg capsules two or three times a day
  Nebulized solution

  - Effective. In some cases may cause hoarseness of voice, oral and pharyngeal candida, tracheal ulceration and asphyxiation. Adrenal suppression in children described

- *Betamethasone valerate* (Bextasol)
  Aerosol 100 μg 1 puff three or four times a day

  - As above

- *Becloforte* useful in chronic severe asthma of children and adults when reduction or withdrawal of oral steroids is desirable

Anticholinergic inhalers : types
'block muscarinic action of acetylcholine'

- *Ipratropium bromide* (Atrovent) 18–36 μg, 1 – 2 puffs two or three times a day.
  - Dry mouth and airways
    Precipitates glaucoma
    Urinary retention

Effective in some when the dose is titrated to suit the patient

Specially useful in wheezy bronchitis

Can be used with β-agonist inhalers ± oral therapy

'Combination' inhalers

- *Fenoterol + ipratropium* (Duovent)

  - Expensive
    Lack of correlation between the amount of each drug.
    Try in 'difficult' cases

- *Salbutamol and beclamethasone* (Ventide)

RESPIRATORY DISEASES

Sodium cromoglycate 'mast-cell stabilizer'	
• Intal and Intal-Co *Spinhaler*, 20 mg up to 8 times a day	• A very powerful prophylactic drug especially in children
Aerosol, 2 mg per 2 puffs – as effective as Spinhaler	• Safe
Nebulizing solution, 1 ml/10 mg 4–6 times daily	• Powdered stuff can irritate the throat
	• Especially effective in extrinsic and exercise induced wheeze
	• Intal-Co indicated in a very few. Isoprenaline may potentiate side-effects as patients are on multiple therapy

Oral drug therapy

Types are

- sympathomimetics
- theophyllines
- steroids
- antihistamines

Sympathomimetics

Sympathomimetics	
• *Salbutamol* Children: 2 mg twice a day. Adults: 4 mg three times a day or *Spandet* – 8 mg once or twice a day. Also available in syrup (for children and very old)	• Spandet particularly useful in patients with early morning 'dip'. Side-effects – as per inhalers
• *Terbutaline* Children 1.5 mg b.d. Adults 5 mg b.d. Also available in syrup.	• Marked tremor in many patients limits its use

BRONCHIAL ASTHMA

Which oral theophylline?

- Regarded as second-line treatment – when inhalers alone are not effective.
- Indicated in patients with wheezy bronchitis.
- Side-effects relatively common (approximately 20%).
- Combination with sympathomimetics may reduce some side-effects. Results of trials suggest additive effect. Hazardous when the dose of β-agonist is high.
- When the dose of theophylline is taken into account – all theophyllines and aminophylline preparations are equally effective.
- Elixirs are absorbed faster than soluble tablets. Useful in children and in acute attacks but less convenient than slow-release preparations for maintenance therapy.
- Rona-slophyllin suitable preparation for children.
- Aminophylline suppositories have no real place in treatment.

Oral steroids

* Use steroid card	
• Prednisone 1 mg, 5 mg. enteric coated 2.5 mg, 5 mg	• Useful in acute severe episodes. 40 mg/day for 1st week then gradually decrease and withdraw after a month
	• Some chronic severe asthmatics may need maintenance dose of 5–7.5 mg/day
	• Side-effects with prolonged therapy – Cushing's syndrome
• Betamethasone, 0.5 mg, dexamethasone	• Not often used in asthma
• Triamcinolone * 1 mg, 2 mg, 4 mg.	• Bruising and proximal mylopathy with long usage. Effective in hay fever, eczema (severe)

Antihistamines

- Useful in seasonal allergic symptoms, e.g. rhinitis.
- Various preparations available.
- Most produce non-tolerable side-effects of drowsiness and lethargy.

- Children do better on them when given a single nocturnal dose, e.g.
  elixir promethazine 20–50 mg/day
  terfenadine tablets
  chlorpheniramine 4 mg twice a day

Nebulizer therapy

- Salbutamol and fenoterol are widely used either as nebules or mixed with saline. Disodium cromoglycate and beclamethasone also available.
- Effective method of administration when oxygen used concurrently (8 l/min).
- Reserved mainly for children and in acute attacks (specially in hospital) when oxygen is readily available.
- Multiflow regulator device necessary over domiciliary oxygen cylinders to provide adequate pressure. These are readily available (approximate cost £70). *Not* prescribed on NHS.

Parenteral therapy

• Hydrocortisone	• In severe asthma give 200 mg by slow i.v. injection. Repeat 6-hourly till improvement occurs following oral prednisone.
• Triamcinolone	• Very useful
	• Given intermittent injections (i.m.) every 3–6 weeks
	• Effective in allergy syndromes
	• May cause bruises, proximal muscle weakness if therapy is prolonged for more than 6 months
	• Hirsutism and menstrual disturbances distressing for the young females
• Depomedrone 40 mg	• Usually effective in children only
• Adrenocorticotrophic hormone (ACTH)	• Rarely used now. May disturb hypothalamic–pituitary function.

CHRONIC SEVERE ASTHMA

- A small percentage of total.
- Very difficult to manage – often needing frequent hospital admissions. They should be referred for a specialist opinion and 'dual-care' appropriate.
- Drug therapy

Nebulized β-agonist	Maintenance	*Oral* or
e.g. salbutamol (nebules)	*inhaled steroids*	*parenteral*
fenoterol	beclomethasone	*steroids* –
Oxygen necessary	e.g. Becotide	triamcinolone is
	Becloforte	EFFECTIVE

- Prognosis relatively poor – often complicated by right heart failure and side-effects of drugs, especially steroids.

ACUTE SEVERE ASTHMA

Whom to refer to hospital?

- *Elderly – often newly diagnosed*. These patients often proceed to respiratory failure (high P_{CO_2} and low P_{O_2}) very rapidly and may need assisted ventilation.
- *A child with 'unstable' disease* especially when there is an 'infective' precipitating cause.
- Presence of cyanosis.
- Presence of *chest pain* (pleuritic) may raise the possibility of *pneumothorax*.
- Those with previous hospital admission especially over the recent period.
- When there are other medical problems, e.g. heart disease, *diabetes mellitus* or *renal disease*.

Acute severe asthma: patients at risk

- Protracted symptoms with no firm diagnosis
- Previous unpredictable and variable clinical course
- Those with marked fall in PEFR in early hours of morning
- Inadvertent use of β-blockers, aspirin and sedatives
- Those with steroid dependent chronic severe asthma in whom therapy is withdrawn abruptly

Features of acute severe asthma

- Tachycardia usually > 110 per min
- Tachypnoea usually > 28 per min
- Pulsus paradoxus usually > 20 mmHg
- Fever ± infection
- Confusion/aggression and anoxia
- Less than 25% of previously best recorded PEFR
- Pneumomediastinum or pneumothorax (chest X-ray)

Management

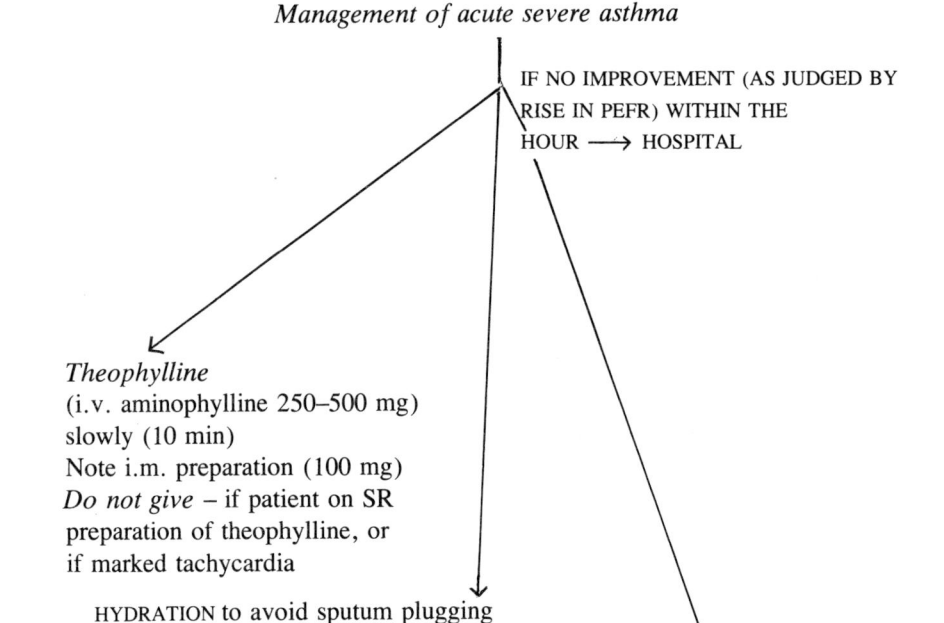

Management of acute severe asthma

IF NO IMPROVEMENT (AS JUDGED BY RISE IN PEFR) WITHIN THE HOUR ⟶ HOSPITAL

Theophylline
(i.v. aminophylline 250–500 mg)
slowly (10 min)
Note i.m. preparation (100 mg)
Do not give – if patient on SR preparation of theophylline, or if marked tachycardia

HYDRATION to avoid sputum plugging
NEBULIZER (preferably with oxygen 8 l/min in most cases)

i.v. hydrocortisone
100 mg stat. Repeat in 6 h.
Oral prednisone:
40 mg/day for 1 week
30 mg/day for 2nd week
20 mg/day for 3rd week
then gradually withdraw

DEATHS FROM ASTHMA

What lessons?

In spite of vigorous 'new' forms of treatment and better health education, there is concern that mortality shows no sign of decline. It has not changed since the mid-1960s[11]. About 1200–1500 deaths are recorded annually in England and Wales. In a prospective study by the British Thoracic Association (BTA) (1979), 82% of deaths had *avoidance* factors *identified – not necessarily* meaning that the deaths could be *prevented*. It is uncertain that management is deficient in those who die as compared to asthmatic patients in general. The BTA (1979) Committee considered that 1:9 deaths were unavoidable.

Unavoidable deaths in asthma

- Sudden severe attack rapidly progressing to death before emergency treatment could be summoned
- Unavoidable delay in summoning help
- Lack of response to treatment already given

Could self-administered sympathomimetic/steroid (parenteral) save those who find themselves in a devastatingly rapid attack leading to death – say within 30 minutes? The problem is: how does one recognize these 'at risk' groups? There are, as yet, no conclusive guidelines. The best one can do is to ensure that most asthmatics are able to record a safe peak flow rate (PEFR) in what they consider a 'quiet' phase. A record greater than 60–65% predicted is acceptable. Therefore there is a need for many asthmatics to monitor their progress at 'home' using a peak flow meter.

Bronchial asthma is omitted as diagnosis in two main groups.

(1) *Those who smoke and cough and wheeze* (it would be easy to label this as chronic bronchitis or wheezy bronchitis). Some patients would 'take' advice from doctors and give up tobacco. Temporarily asthmatics will deteriorate and wheeze more – a clear indication that asthma can coexist with bronchitis. These patients should receive 'full' bronchodilator therapy.

(2) *Children*. In a study[12] the diagnosis of asthma was made in only 14 of 87 children who had had four to 12 or more episodes of wheezing a year; less than a third of the children received a bronchodilator. Fifty per cent of the children had lost more than 50 days off school.

The BTA (1979) study also recognized many deaths in asthma where diagnosis was not made (majority were labelled chronic bronchitis). It is wise to adopt a high index of suspicion and 'think asthma'. There is no harm in 'overtreating' a wheezy patient (especially a child) when other conditions have been excluded.

RESPIRATORY DISEASES

Who at risk?

- Early (childhood) onset
- Long history > 20 years
- Chronic disability
- Short admissions < 3 months
- Females > 45 years
- Unstable state (on PEFR)

It is difficult to convince many that the 'asthma deaths' in the 1960s were not related to overuse of inhalers. The BTA (1979) study and various other investigators have shown conclusively that undertreatment remains a problem and there is no evidence that excessive medication contributed to deaths.

Supervision by GPs of asthmatic patients was regarded adequate in only two of 90 patients (BTA 1979 study); more frequent follow-up in 70, deterioration not appreciated quick enough in 57. Nineteen cases failed to obtain continuity in care (seen by various practitioners)

GPs said

50% of patients took therapy

50% 'non-compliant'

GPs should

See 'at risk' patients frequently and at a short notice

Frequent PEFR

Early referral in difficult cases

SUMMARY: PROTOCOLS OF CARE

Children

Majority of children will have persistent cough and wheeze at night. Other allergic symptoms of rhinitis/conjunctivitis/eczema. A small group will have nasal polyps and exercise-induced wheeze.

Do

- PEFR several times a day
- Allergy tests (PETS)
- Chest X-ray in severe cases to exclude eosinophilic infiltrates
- ENT confirmation of nasal polyps. Surgical removal not necessary.

BRONCHIAL ASTHMA

Give

- Sympathomimetic (salbutamol or terbutaline) inhaler
- Add { sodium cromoglycate ± beclomethasone if strong allergic basis and exercise worsening symptoms
- Antihistamine elixir (at night) when eczema, rhinitis and hay fever
- Hyposensitization when IgE levels very high
- Oral theophyllines, sympathomimetics and steroids in a few chronic cases
- Hydrocortisone in severe attacks
- Nebulized therapy in a very few (obtain specialist opinion)

Young adults

Young adults may give previous history of asthma, wheezy bronchitis, eczema and hay fever. Exercise-induced wheeze likely. Will find difficulty in sports with reduction in exercise tolerance.

Do

- PEFR several times a day
- Allergy tests in selected few
- Chest X-ray if diagnosis in doubt

Give

- *Sympathomimetic* inhaler (salbutamol, terbutaline, rimiterol) as a prophylaxis
- Beclomethasone (inhaled) during exacerbation and in moderately severe chronic symptoms
- *Antihistamines and hyposensitization not necessary*
- Oral *theophyllines, sympathomimetics* in exacerbations
- *Oral steroids* effective in short courses
- *Hydrocortisone* in severe symptoms
- *Nebulizer* inconvenient and *not* effective
- Short course of *triamcinolone* injection in selected 'allergic' cases

Middle-aged

Middle-aged asthmatics – some will give previous/family history. Occupational aetiology? Experience 'tightness' of chest with wheeze. Some nocturnal symptoms of wheeze and cough. Often a non-smoker.

Do

- PEFR (demonstrate reversibility)
- 'Challenge' tests if occupation relevant
- Chest X-ray necessary to exclude other disorders especially in a smoker
- Cardiac assessment (including e.c.g.)

Give

- *Sympathomimetic inhaler* (salbutamol, terbutaline) as prophylaxis
- Beclomethasone on regular basis
- Oral *sympathomimetics* or *theophyllines* in some severe chronic cases and in exacerbation
- Oral prednisone in short courses in exacerbation and in acute cases. Maintenance dose in a very few cases
- Hydrocortisone in status asthmaticus
- Triamcinolone (i.m.) when prednisone therapy has failed

Elderly

Elderly asthmatics may present for the first time. Attacks proceed rapidly to severe life-threatening situation. Always a non-smoker. 'Stress' may be a factor. The mild to moderate chronic cases will find limitation of exercise tolerance, difficulty in sleeping – confining the patient to the house. Often misdiagnosed as chronic bronchitis, emphysema and heart disease.

Do

- PEFR (note reversibility after 'trial' of therapy)
- Chest X-ray to exclude other disorders
- Cardiac assessment (including e.c.g.)

Give

- *Inhalers 'tolerated' by very few*. Nebulized therapy may be more appropriate
- Oral *theophyllines and sympathomimetics:* start with 'small' doses
- Many will need *maintenance oral steroids* and often very effective. Ignore the likelihood of side-effects in favour of improvement of quality of life
- Death in *acute* attacks high. Refer to hospital for treatment

References

1. Clark, T. J. H. and Godfrey, S. (eds) (1983). *Epidemiology in Asthma* (London: Chapman & Hall)
2. Pepys, J. (1967). Hypersensitivity to inhaled organic antigens. *J. R. Coll. Phys.* **2,** 42–8
3. Martin, A. J. *et al.* (1980). *Br. Med. J.,* **280,** 1391
4. Godfrey, S. (1983). The wheezy infant. In *Recent Advances in Paediatrics, No 7,* (Edinburgh and London: Churchill Livingstone)
5. Editorial (1981). Asthma – a challenge for general practice. *J. R. Coll. Gen. Pract.,* **31,** 323–4
6. Anderson, H. R. *et al.* (1980) *Br. Med. J.,* **281,** 1190–4
7. Death from asthma in two regions in England. *Br. Med. J.* 1982, **285,** 1251–5
8. Speight, A. N. P. (1978). Is childhood asthma being underdiagnosed: *Br. Med. J.,* **2,** 331–2
9. Dekker, E. and Groen, J. (1956). *J. Psychosom. Res.,* **1,** 58–67
10. Paterson, J. W. *et al.* (1979). *Am. Rev. Resp. Dis.,* **120,** 1149–88
11. Editorial (1979). Deaths from asthma. *Br. Med. J.,* **1,** 1520
12. Speight, A. N. P. *et al.* (1983). *Br. Med. J.,* **286,** 1253–6

7

Tumours of the lung

☐ ☐ ☐ ☐ ☐ ☐ ☐ ☐ ☐ ☐ ☐ ☐

WHAT ARE THEY ?

Types

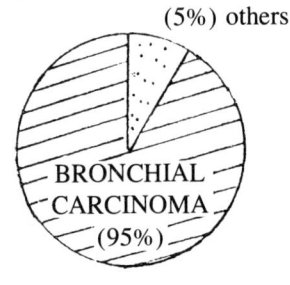

BRONCHIAL CARCINOMA (95%)
(5%) others

70 tumours or tumour-like conditions reported occurring in the lungs or pleura[1]

Others

- *Adenoma* ('carcinoid' or 'cylindromata')
  < 1%

- *Secondary carcinoma*
  < 1% from kidney, prostate thyroid, choriocarcinoma

- *Alveolar cell carcinoma*
  < 0.5%

- *Mesothelioma, lymphoma (including Hodgkin's)*
  < 1%

- Rare: *Hamartoma: lipoma*

Features

- Suspect in a young patient with haemoptysis, diarrhoea, flushing and wheezing

- No definite respiratory symptoms. Pain, haemoptysis late

- Diffuse lung shadowing. Difficult to diagnose on CXR

- Patient seriously ill

- Incidental finding

SIGNIFICANCE

- Bronchial carcinoma is by far the commonest of the group (95% of total). Also known as 'carcinoma of bronchus' or 'carcinoma of lung'.
- A general practitioner may see only one or two new cases of bronchial carcinoma per year. Physicians in local district hospitals may be referred up to 200 new cases per year. Therefore misconception may exist.
- In 80% of cases referred to hospital, the general practitioners would have suspected or already made the diagnosis.
- A chest X-ray suggesting bronchogenic carcinoma can sometimes mislead (see differential diagnosis of such an opacity, Ch.3). Need for histological confirmation.
- Bronchial carcinoma is the most common cancer in *males* and third commonest in *females*. It is likely – if present trends continue – lung cancer will be more common than breast cancer in females in the next 5 years.
- Only 6–8% of males and 8–12% of females will be alive 5 years after the diagnosis – irrespective of the choice of treatment used.
- Recognition and treatment of the disease while it is still localized increases the overall 5-year survival to about 15–20%.

CAUSAL FACTORS

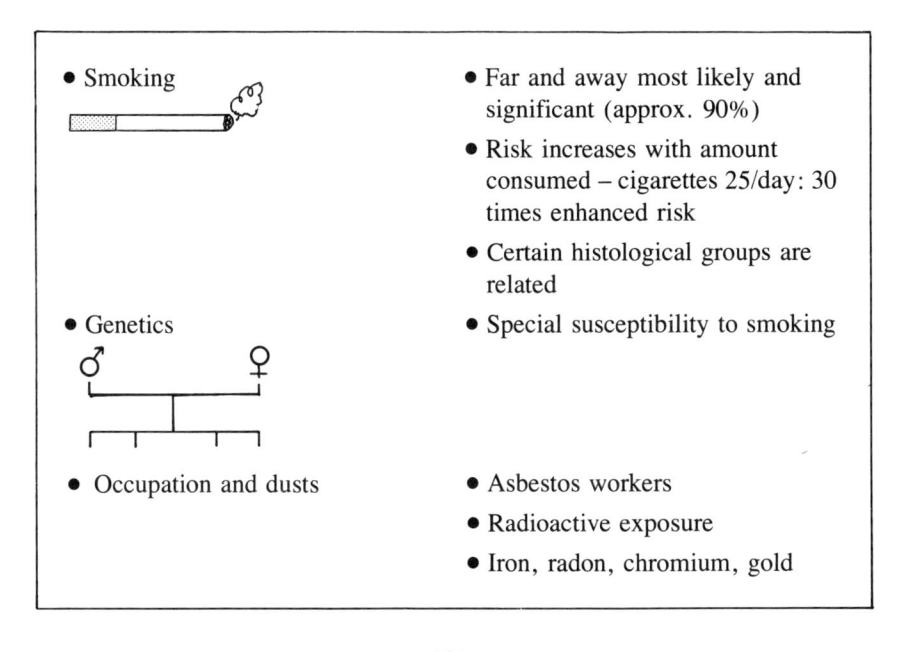

• Smoking	• Far and away most likely and significant (approx. 90%)
	• Risk increases with amount consumed – cigarettes 25/day: 30 times enhanced risk
	• Certain histological groups are related
• Genetics	• Special susceptibility to smoking
• Occupation and dusts	• Asbestos workers
	• Radioactive exposure
	• Iron, radon, chromium, gold

RESPIRATORY DISEASES

*Deaths per 100 000 population – comparison with other respiratory disorders; all ages**

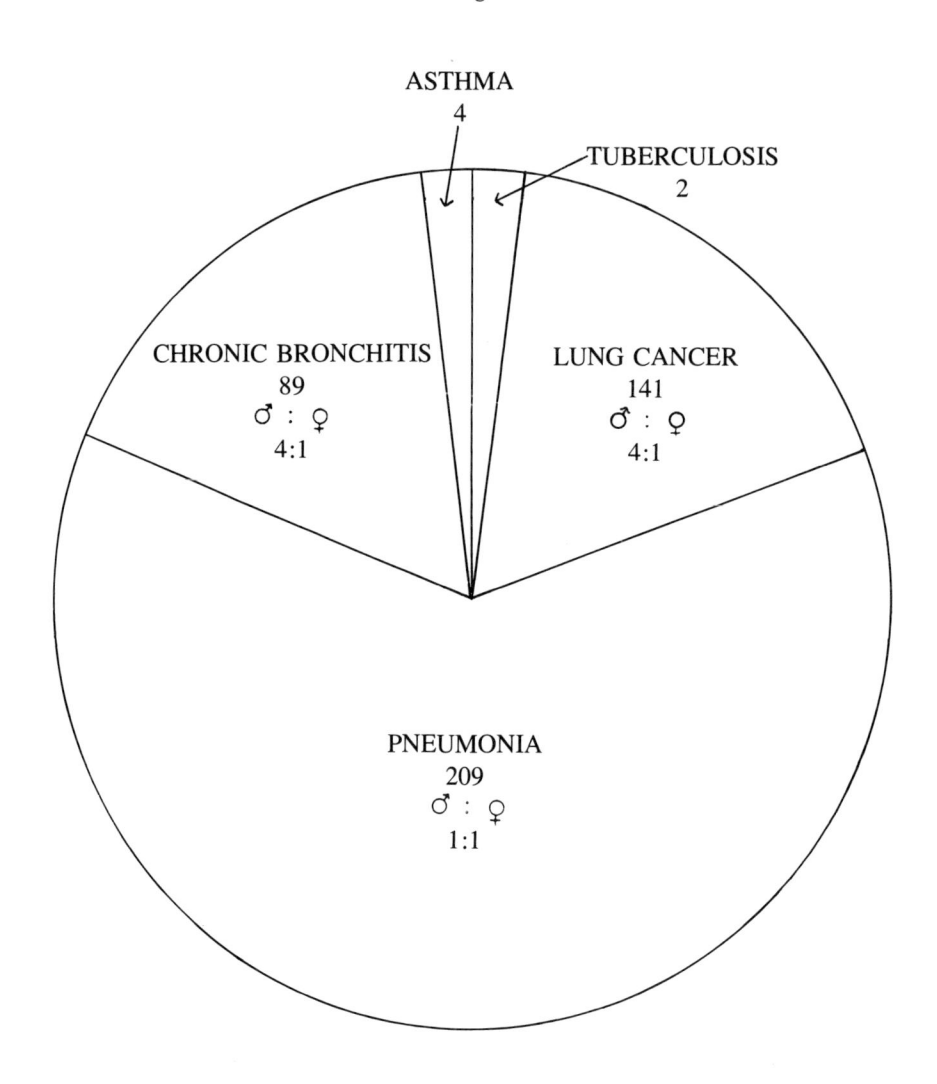

ASTHMA
4

TUBERCULOSIS
2

CHRONIC BRONCHITIS
89
♂ : ♀
4:1

LUNG CANCER
141
♂ : ♀
4:1

PNEUMONIA
209
♂ : ♀
1:1

*Office of Population Censuses & Surveys 1971

CLINICAL FEATURES – RELATED TO HISTOLOGICAL GROUPS

Squamous cell (epidermoid)

- 35–50% of the total
- ♂ : ♀ = 10 : 3
- Strong relation to smoking
- Slow growing
- Metastases relatively late – primarily to hilar nodes
- Radiology:

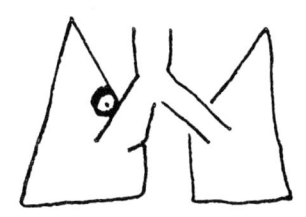

Central – often cavitated

- Likely to be resectable if early diagnosis

Special feature:
- Hypercalcaemia
  (will respond to prednisone and treatment of underlying tumour)
- *Survival* (5 years) : 28%[2]

Small cell (anaplastic) – oat cell

- 25–30% of the total
- ♂ : ♀ = 3 : 1
- Related to smoking
- Very rapid growth
- Very early spread to mediastinum and distally
- Radiology:

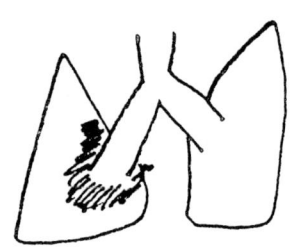

Hilar with secondaries

- Resectability – poor

Special feature:
- Excess ACTH (Cushing's), ADH (inappropriate)

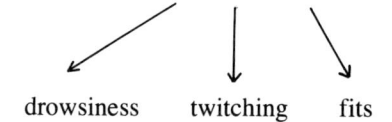

     drowsiness twitching fits

- *Survival* (5 years) : 5%

Adenocarcinoma

- 15–20% of the total
- ♂ = ♀
- No definite relation to smoking
    (special risk in scar tissue due to asbestosis)
- Intermediate growth and spread
- Radiology:

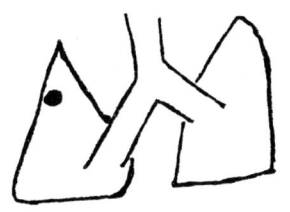

Peripheral lesion < 4 cm

- Resectability – poor

Special feature:
- Complicated TB and asbestos scars
- *Survival* (5 years): 17%

Large cell anaplastic

- 10–15% of the total
- ♂ : ♀ = 2 : 1
- Related to smoking
- Rapidly growing
- Early spread
- Radiology:

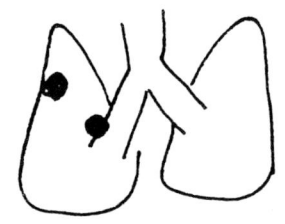

Variable: peripheral or central

- Resectability – poor

Special feature:
- Painful gynaecomastia
- *Survival* (5 years): 15%

MANAGEMENT

This is divided into the following:
- Early diagnosis
- Initial assessment and investigations
- Selection of patients to be referred to a specialist
- What categories of treatments available
- Treatment of troublesome symptoms
- Terminal care

Diagnosis

- Bronchial carcinoma in its 'early' stages may produce no significant symptoms or signs.
- A 'typical' patient would be a middle-aged smoker – of either sex – with about 6 weeks' history of
(1) Weight loss of >6 kg
(2) Cough (insidious and distressing)
(3) Breathlessness
(4) Haemoptysis and chest pain
- Examination may often be normal. In more advanced disease, the following may be seen:
    finger and toe clubbing ($+$ nicotine-staining)
    lymph nodes (supraclavicular fossae and axillae)
    stridor and monophonic wheeze
    hepatomegaly $\pm$ ascites
    gynaecomastia $\pm$ arthropathy
    thromboembolism (migrans)

RESPIRATORY DISEASES

Unusual presentation

- *Hoarse voice*

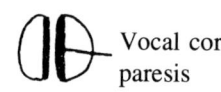

    Vocal cord paresis

- Signifies recurrent laryngeal nerve involvement. May be confirmed on laryngoscopy or bronchoscopy

- *Pleural effusion*

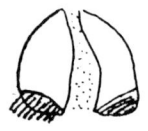

    Large unilateral/ bilateral effusion

- Secondary involvement. Aspiration ± pleural biopsy necessary for diagnosis and relief of breathlessness. Intrapleural chemotherapy useful

- *Pericardial effusion*

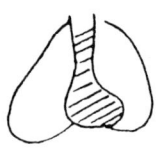

    Disseminated disease. Could lead to difficulties in diagnosis

- Either as a direct invasion or secondary to severe heart failure. TB has to be excluded

- *Skin disorders*

- Many, including:
    dermatomyositis
    acanthosis nigrans
    metastatic nodules

- *Nervous system involvement*

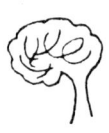

    No evidence of cerebral metastases in many, i.e. para-malignant disorders (PMD)

- Cerebellar degeneration: ataxia, falls.
- Eaton-Lambert syndrome: 'myasthenic' (e.m.g. useful).
- Motor neuron disease

- *Endocrine complications*

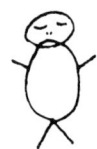

    Cushing's. 'Moans, groans and stones'; ↑ Ca

- ADH oversecretion (confusion, fits, drowsiness):
- ACTH ⟶ Cushing's
- hypercalcaemia

Assessment and investigations

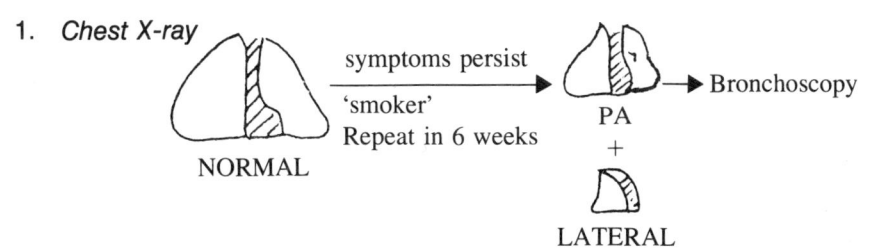

1. *Chest X-ray*

NORMAL → symptoms persist, 'smoker', Repeat in 6 weeks → PA + LATERAL → Bronchoscopy

This is essential. If the initial film is reported normal and symptoms persist – especially in a smoker – a further film should be undertaken in about 6–8 weeks including on this occasion an appropriate lateral film. A normal chest X-ray does not exclude a lesion conclusively and therefore in a patient with continuing symptoms a specialist opinion will be necessary.

> *NORMAL CXR*
> Does not exclude diagnosis

A significant proportion (approximately 5–7%) with normal chest X-ray and sputa examination – a diagnosis of bronchial carcinoma will be made on bronchoscopy/mediastinoscopy.

RESPIRATORY DISEASES

Chest X-ray findings (common)
(Primary : secondary carcinoma)

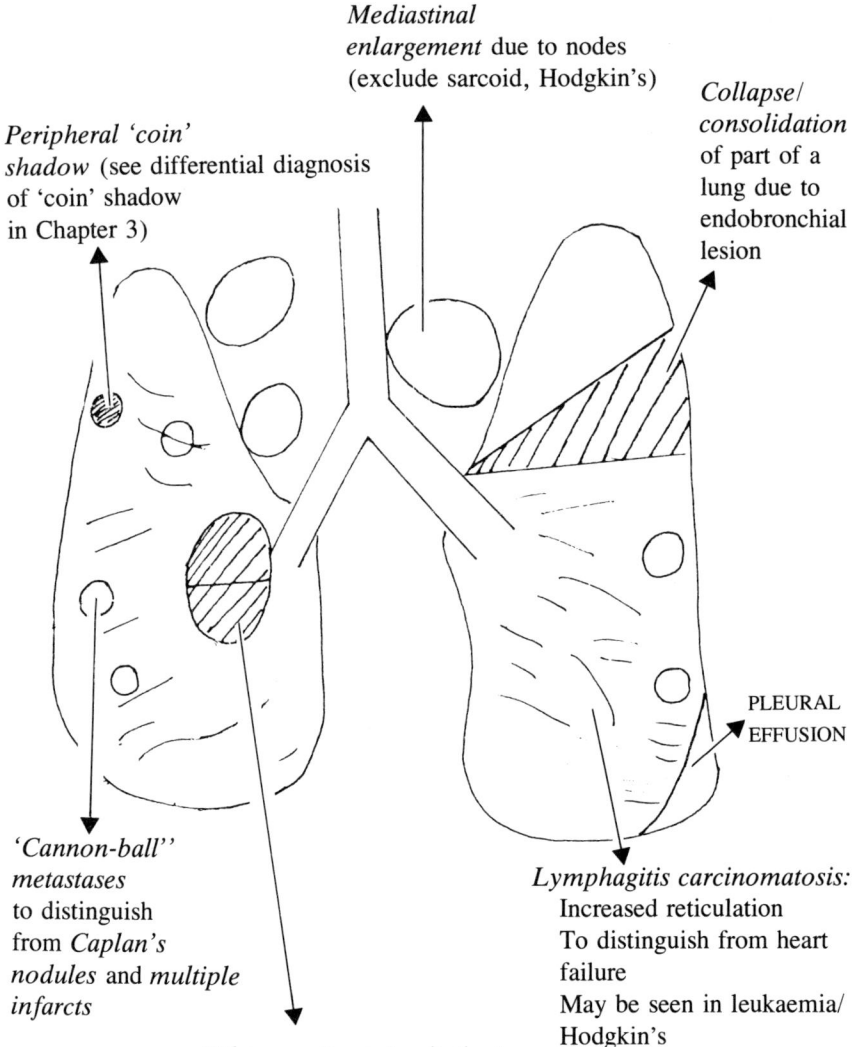

Peripheral 'coin' shadow (see differential diagnosis of 'coin' shadow in Chapter 3)

Mediastinal enlargement due to nodes (exclude sarcoid, Hodgkin's)

Collapse/ consolidation of part of a lung due to endobronchial lesion

PLEURAL EFFUSION

'Cannon-ball' metastases to distinguish from *Caplan's nodules* and *multiple infarcts*

Lymphagitis carcinomatosis: Increased reticulation
To distinguish from heart failure
May be seen in leukaemia/Hodgkin's

Hilar opacity ± (cavitating): Difficulty in distinguishing from prominent vascular (hilar) shadows
Tomogram may help

2. *Examination of sputum*

Three separate specimens are necessary and should be sent (*in proper containers* – available from histopathology laboratories) for *cytology*. Incidence of *false positive* is very *small*. When the laboratory is in 'doubt' – further specimens should be sent. Cytological examination of gastric aspirate is not indicated.

3. *Tuberculin test*

A tuberculin test (1:1000) dilution should be undertaken in patients especially when the chest X-ray suggests upper lobe consolidation. In these patients sputa for AAFB may also be necessary. A negative tuberculin test is regarded as a poor prognostic index for bronchial carcinoma.

4. *FEV_1, FVC*

Where facilities are available, a FEV_1 (forced expiratory volume), *FVC* (forced vital capacity) may help. Those with $FEV_1 > 1.6$ litres may carry a better prognosis (*see* surgical management sections, *below*).

5. *Biopsy*

Where *lymph nodes* are palpable and *histological confirmation* is necessary, biopsy (through a needle) is safe and effective in diagnosis. The procedure could be undertaken by a pathologist (patient visiting hospital for the procedure only – as a day case). Many laboratories allow general practitioners to borrow such aspiration biopsy sets.

Whom to refer to hospital

- Majority of patients (> 85%) could be diagnosed conclusively in general practice – good history, examination, chest X-ray (PA and lateral) and sputa cytology.
- The general practitioner may wish to treat at home ± hospice those with severe disease (including dissemination; the very old).
- Relatives or patient of some chosen for 'home care' may request a 'second opinion'. This should not be denied.
- Those without family support may be difficult to treat at home.
- Some chosen for home care will eventually need intensive nursing (usually in a medical ward in hospital) *or* advice regarding support and pain-control from the hospice. Early involvement of physician/hospice team is indicated.

RESPIRATORY DISEASES

'Urgent' referral

Indications

- A *localized lung lesion* – in a well-looking individual. Histology – *squamous cell*.
- Persistent 'heavy' *haemoptyses*.
- *Severe pain* (either due to the lesion or rib involvement).
  Pancoat's tumour is an apical lesion involving the rib and brachial plexus.
- *Stridor* (inspiratory wheeze) may mean upper respiratory tract obstruction due to glands.
- *Severe breathlessness*. This may be due to impending main bronchus obstruction or pleural effusion.
- *Paramalignant syndrome* (PMD), e.g.
  inappropriate ADH secretion
  cerebellar degeneration
  Cushing's/diabetes mellitus/thyrotoxicosis
  hypertrophic pulmonary osteoarthropathy (HPOA)

How to seek an urgent appointment (assuming diagnosis is made)

- It is not necessary for a physician to assess 'operability' and patients with *localized lesion* should be referred to a *thoracic surgeon* – especially when the finding of tumour is incidental.
- Patients with *haemoptyses* may have an operable cavitating lesion but should be referred to a physician (with bronchoscopy facilities) for further assessment and advice.
- Those with severe bony pain, SVC obstruction, breathlessness, stridor and paramalignant syndromes should be regarded as *medical emergencies* and must be assessed and treated in hospital at least in the initial period. Many will benefit from palliative radiotherapy. It is likely that the condition will be advanced here.

Further investigations:	*'Hospital cases'*

• Radiology	• Tomography
	    may reveal cavitation and calcification (TB)
	    typical appearance is of an irregular mass with 'sun-ray' projections
	    screening of diaphragm movement

• Image scanning	• Liver, brain, bone scan to exclude metastases

• 'Blood tests'	• Normocytic normochromic anaemia and high ESR do *not* necessarily signify poor prognosis.
	    Abnormal electrolytes including Ca^{2+} indicate paramalignant disorders
	    High alkaline phosphatase – in pathological fractures and liver secondaries

• Electrocardiograph	• To exclude incidental heart disease. Conduction defects may be seen
• Lung function tests	• Measurement of transfer factor to exclude interstitial lung involvement
• Bronchoscopy/thoracoscopy and mediastinoscopy	• Diagnosis and assessing operability

Categories of treatment

- Surgical
- Chemotherapy/immunotherapy
- Radiotherapy/laser
- Supportive

Choice of therapy for a particular patient depends upon:
- the clinical background (including patient's preference after discussion)
- the histological type
- TNM classification (*see* table below)

TNM categories of bronchial carcinoma*

Primary tumours (T)
T1 Tumour < 3 cm diameter
T2 Tumour > 3 cm diameter
T3 Tumour any size

Regional lymph nodes (N)
N0 No nodes
N1 Peribronchial and/or ipsilateral hilar nodes
N2 Mediastinal nodes

Distant metastases (M)
M0 No distant metastases
M1 Distant metastases

From: American Joint Committee (1974)

Bronchial carcinoma
Survival (%) at 2 years and staging categories*

	Squamous	Adeno-carcinoma	Large cell	Small cell
Stage 1 T1 N0 M0 T1 N1 M0 T2 N0 M0	47	46	43	6
Stage 2 T2 N1 M0	40	14	13	5
Stage 3 T3 any N or M N2 any T or M M1 any T or N	11	8	13	3

From: Mountain *et al.* (1974). *Am. J. Roentgenol. Rad. Ther. Nucl. Med.*, **120**, 131.8

Long survival following surgical treatment requires complete removal of tumour. Staging is therefore important. Histology is less important if 'curative' procedure possible. Five-year survival in this group (squamous/adenocarcinoma/large cell) averages 25%[3]. In more advanced disease, histology becomes of significance – because of its metastatic potential.

Most surgeons prefer to preserve as much normal lung tissue as possible and therefore lobectomy is preferred to any other procedure. Surgical mortality is twice as high in pneumonectomy.

Patients with small cell cancer are surgical proposition only when presenting with a small, peripheral, asymptomatic nodule.

Those with chest wall or rib cage involvement could be candidates for *en bloc* resection. Some will need preoperative radiation therapy.

Surgery

Types of procedures

Thoracotomy (entry into the chest at the level of 5th rib)

- Lobectomy (most common)
- Pneumonectomy
- Segmental or wedge resection
- Sleeve resection

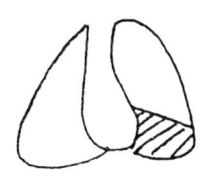

Lobectomy
Removal of part of a lobe or lung and affected, identifiable nodes. The nodes may be hilar or mediastinal ± heart and chest wall involvement may make the case 'inoperable'

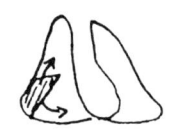

On the right side the middle lobe removed with either upper or lower lobe depending on involvement at the horizontal/oblique fissure

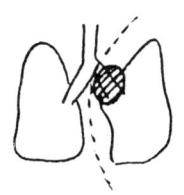

Pneumonectomy

A central lesion involving the main bronchus

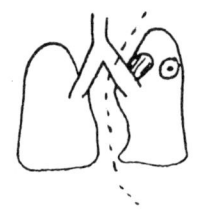

A peripheral lesion with hilar nodes

Segmental or wedge resection

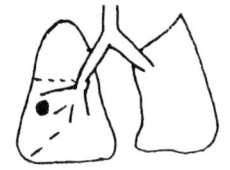

Well defined resection in a localized lesion
Uncommon procedure in lung cancer

Sleeve resection

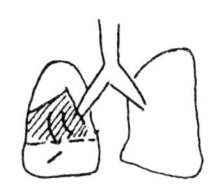

When the left or right upper lobe orifice is involved, rings of the bronchi are removed with the lobe and the remaining 'bits' repaired by anastomosis. This spares the patient a pneumonectomy

Further 'difficult' variations include
Radical resection in Pancoat's tumour

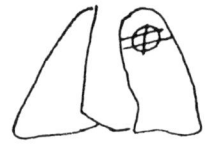

'Clearance' of mediastinal space (nodes) ± heart involvement

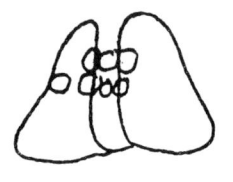

Patients likely to do well:

- Carcinoma *in situ*.
- A tumour <3 cm in diameter, without pleural spread or distant metastases. If lymph nodes involved, confined to same side.
- A tumour >3 cm but no pleural, nodal or distant involvement.

What problems (post-thoracotomy): immediate and late

Problems	Features
Pain	• Encourages collapse of the healthy lung
	• Can be relieved – for a short period by intercostal nerve block
	• Regular, adequate postoperative analgesia necessary in most
Infection (depressed immunity, smoking habit, pain and previous lung disease enhance the risks)	• Antibiotics
	• Physiotherapy
	• Regular suction
	• Relief of pain
Pulmonary infarction/embolism	• ? Help to give prophylactic s.c. heparin
	• Early diagnosis and treatment important
Cardiac (risks greater in less fit, 'old' patients who need pneumonectomy)	• Arrythmias and infarction likely
	• Diagnose early and treat appropriately
Wound pain (this is the one likely to involve the GP commonly). Known to occur in 5–10% of patients	• Give regular analgesics (aspirin, paracetamol)
	• Add non-steroid anti-inflammatory agents
	• Transcutaneous nerve stimulator (obtain from 'pain' clinics)
	• Sodium valproate (Epilim) and carbamazepine (Tegretol) worth trying
	• Get advice from the surgeon and anaesthetist

Other complications

- *Empyema thoracis*

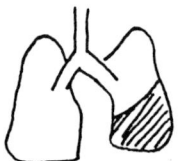

    (risk worse following pneumonectomy)

- *Bronchopleural fistula*

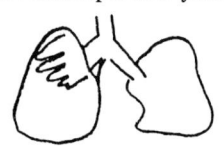

    due to problems at the 'stump' site or recurrence of tumour

- Risk when infection pre-exists in the lung (preoperative), e.g. abscess cavity with the cancer
- Organisms

    Anaerobes
    Gram-positive cocci

- The effusion is drained dry and antibiotics installed. The process may need to be repeated
- Rarely decortication
- Haemoptysis, cough, debility
- Bronchoscopic assessment

Postoperative survival of lung cancer

Favourable	Unfavourable
• Age < 60 years	• Age > 60 years
• Right lung involved	• Left lung involved (aortic arch interferes in operation)
• Lobectomy	• Pneumonectomy
• No associated pulmonary disease (*Normal* preop lung scan)	• Associated pulmonary disease (abnormal preop lung scan)
• No other medical disorders, e.g. heart disease, diabetes, hypertension	• Presence of other medical disorders
• Weight loss < 6 kg	• Weight loss > 6 kg
• Squamous cell	• Other histological types with hilar, mediastinal nodal involvement
• Non-smoker	• Smoker

Development of second primary : postoperative

Those undergoing 'curative' surgery have been compared with age-matched male samples[4]. For at least 8 years postoperatively the surgically treated lung cancer patients had a significantly greater risk of death. Highest risk in the first year ($\times 8$), lowest by the seventh year ($\times 2$). Most deaths were due to recurrent disease – some due to a second primary lesion. Estimated 1:5 may develop a second primary.

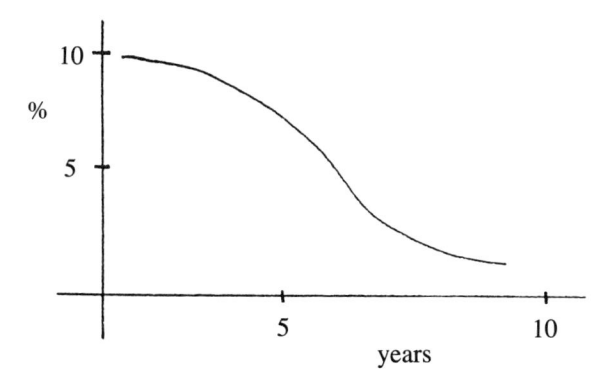

Risks of a second primary

For surgical treatment (summary)

- A young patient < 65 years
- Asymptomatic peripheral nodule (irrespective of histology)
- TMN stage 1
- Good lung function tests
- A normal lung scan
- Absence of other pulmonary/extrapulmonary disorder

Chemotherapy

- Use limited as uncertainty in response and very significant side-effects of drugs used.
- Majority of chemotherapeutic agents have to be administered intravenously.
- As yet no consensus as to what drug combinations to use and for what cancers.

Indications

- Certain small cell tumours (non-small cell show *no* benefit)
- Malignant pleural effusions
- Adjuvant to surgery and radiotherapy

Small cell carcinoma

This tumour disseminates readily and will often present with systemic manifestations. It is most responsive to chemotherapeutic agents (response rate 20–30%). Combination drugs preferred to a single agent. About two thirds of the patients may obtain relief of pain, cough, breathlessness, haemoptysis and SVC obstruction. However, median survival is less than 1 year. Absence of paramalignant disorders, e.g. inappropriate ADH secretion, offer a better response to treatment. It is favoured that patients should be assessed for and treated with chemotherapeutic agents in hospital. However, a GP will deal with many of the side-effects of these drugs. He will have to decide if these are due to the drugs or underlying disease.

Drugs commonly used

A combination of 2/3/4 is preferred.

- Cyclophosphamide
    Oral 50–100 mg daily
    i.v. 100–500 mg (depending on regimen)
- Vincristine
    i.v. 1–5 mg/day
- Methotrexate
    Oral 2.5–10 mg weekly
    i.v. 25 mg weekly (depending on regimen)
- Epipodophyllotoxin
    oral 100 mg b.d. for 5 days at 4 weeks and 6 weeks
    injection 20 mg/ml to be diluted
- Doxorubicin
    i.v. up to 100 mg/day

Anti-cancer drugs

What problems?

- Often difficult to decide whether the new symptoms related to the underlying cancer or the drugs.

- Where a GP is unfamiliar with the drug – the patient should be referred back to 'the specialist' unit and the GP should ask for information pertaining to the special drugs.
- The GP may wish to discuss with the patient and relatives if, in the light of the problems, the treatment programme should be continued, especially in advanced disease.
- If 'the specialist' proposes to continue treatment – especially when objective response has occurred – he may wish to 'keep' the patient in hospital for the whole length of treatment.

Management of side-effects

Nausea and vomiting

- Feature of most anti-cancer drugs
- Accompanied by anorexia and weight loss
- Advise patient to take small meals frequently
- Give metoclopramide oral or i.m. regularly, chlorpromazine and domperidone may help ± antacids

Hair-loss

- A particular problem with vinca alkaloids and etoposide
- Very important to warn the patient before starting treatment
- Occurs in 3–4 weeks
- A wig will need to be ordered
- In some, hair regrows quite quickly

Marrow toxicity

- Leukopenia/thrombocytopenia could be devastating, leading to infection/haemorrhage. Look in the mouth and eyes for evidence of haemorrhage
- Occurs after 2 weeks and improves in 3 weeks
- Refer back to Oncology Unit. Patient may need red cells and platelet replacement ± antibiotics

---

Mouth ulcers

- Often painful
- Lesions in pharynx and oesophagus particularly troublesome. Encourage fluids
- Give amphotericin B (Fungilin) and nystatin lozenges regularly
- Orabase (gelatin paste) and lignocaine lozenges or paste may help

---

Other problems

- *Local cellulitis/thrombophlebitis*
  Treat conservatively. Analgesics ± poultice
- *Lung changes*
  Increase in breathlessness and change on chest X-ray.
  Bleomycin, busulphan and methotrexate more likely.
  Give large doses of prednisone (45 mg/day) and inform the Oncology Unit
- *Cardiotoxicity*
  Heart failure and conduction defects – specially with adriamycin. Drug will need to be withdrawn
- *Peripheral neuropathy*
  May be reversible. In some may result in severe disability

Management of malignant pleural effusions

- Advanced disease may be complicated by pleural and peritoneal effusions – causing breathlessness, debility and abdominal pain.
- Quality of life could be improved by aspirations (often repeated) and installation of chemotherapeutic agents.

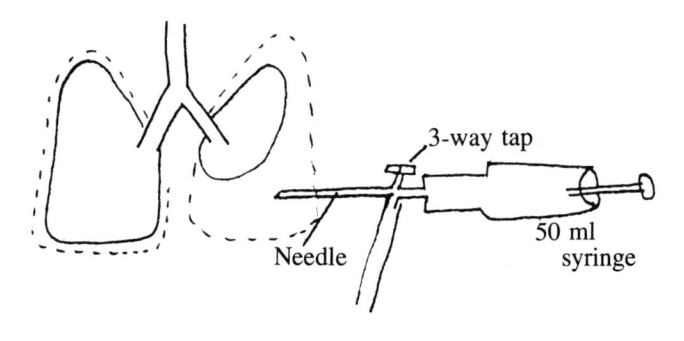

Complications

Pneumothorax
Empyema } therefore repeat chest X-ray after aspiration.
Air embolism

Drugs used

Tetracycline, 1–4 g, in the pleural space may prevent reaccumulation. Procedure painful, therefore give adequate analgesics.

Cyclophosphamide 50–100 mg.

Bleomycin 15–60 mg in 100 ml of saline (alkylating agent).

Chemotherapy adjuvant to surgery and radiotherapy

Radiation therapy may be used to decrease or eradicate large tumour masses and to sterilize tumour in areas where chemotherapy finds sanctuary, e.g. brain. Otherwise there is no evidence so far that chemotherapy used as adjuvant to surgery or radiotherapy is of any significant benefit.

Immunotherapy

Cancer of lung causes immunosuppression as indicated by T-lymphocyte counts and is most manifest in metastatic disease. Those patients who retain immune reactivity have a slightly better prognosis. Trials of *intrapleural BCG organisms* are still continuing. *Levamisole* is also in its 'infant' stage of evaluation.

Radiotherapy

Indications

- Curative intent (localized treatment for localized disease).
- Palliation (relief of symptoms).

Results of trials: choice of patient

- *For non-small cell carcinoma*, surgery preferred to radiation in operable cases.
- *For small cell carcinoma*, neither surgery nor radiation therapy alone is optimal for the majority and *chemotherapy* should be included in treatment programme.
- There is a place for radiation as a 'curative' therapy in locally unresectable but non-metastasized lesion (squamous cell).

'Palliative' treatment

- Relief of *pain* either from the lesion, bony metastases (Pancoat's syndrome), soft tissue deposits, cerebral secondaries or hypertrophic osteoarthropathy (HPOA).
- Control of *haemoptysis*.
- Relief of *breathlessness*. Reduction in the size of tumour may prevent collapse of whole or part of a lung.
- *Irradiation* of tumour may temporarily alleviate paramalignant syndromes including inappropriate ADH secretion, ACTH secretion; gynaecomastia, thromboembolism.

Supportive therapy

Management of troublesome symptoms is summarized in the following tables. For further details see Chapter 8, on management of terminal illness.

Management of troublesome symptoms

• *Cough* often dry, painful, worse at night	• Will respond when the underlying tumour is treated • In presence of advanced disease use: 　'Brompton' mixture containing morphine 5–20 mg 4–6-hourly Methadone 5–10 ml two or four times a day

• *Haemoptysis* (slight in early stages, often painless) – as a result of cavitation of the lesion	• In advanced cases radiation will help • When very heavy – oral iron and blood transfusion necessary • Ethamsylate 500 mg b.d. may help

• *Bone-pains* (constant, severe distress) Back pain from spinal metastases – may proceed to paraplegia. Seek a medical or neurosurgical opinion)	• Usually due to metastases • Localized radiotherapy especially in Pancoat's • Adequate analgesics – including morphine • A good diet

• *Breathlessness* This may be due to: collapse of the lung pleural effusion: aspirate cardiac involvement debility pain	• Relieve pain • Give prednisone 5–10 mg two or three times a day • Oxygen: domiciliary

• *Debility* This is invariable with advanced disease	• Encourage a higher food intake ± alcohol, 'small' meals (appetizing) taken frequently • Give prednisone and vitamins

• *Anxiety/restlessness and depression:*   common features   occasionally as a result of   perceiving the importance of   illness
 	
In a study[5] 74 diagnosed but undisclosed:
  88% either knew or suspected
  14% wanted to know
  32% wanted their diagnosis confirmed
  none wanted to know whether they will 'live' or 'die'
	• 'Talk out' patient's fears and worries
	• Involve hospice/clergy
	• Relieve pain
	• Anxiolytic drugs like diazepam, lorazepam and flupenthixol of help
	• Psychiatrist *not* necessary

- *General nursing*
  debility and wasting causes oral thrush, impaction and trophic ulcers
- Most relatives incapable of managing all
- 'Practice' nurses and hospice team should be involved if hospital admission not indicated

Social aspects and terminal care

Bronchial carcinoma is still generating a lot of *misunderstanding* in management, ignorance of its aetiology and *erroneous beliefs* as to its 'cure' potential. If cancer education in the lay public is to succeed, the educationalists need to be better 'informed'.

Should the patient be told? A cancer patient who feels he is 'not being told enough', is not necessarily asking for the truth, but is very often seeking greater professional attention, more sympathetic care, and information about what to expect in the immediate future. Many on hearing the truth have no option but to come to terms with the cold, factual reality, even though they may be psychologically incapable of doing so.

Patients' reactions to their diagnosis [6]

	Male	Female	Total %
Approval	61	92	66.2
Denial that they had been told	23	21	19.0
Disapproval	0	17	7.4
Inconclusive	9	8	7.4

- There are over 150 terminal care teams in UK.
- Many will work closely with their 'local' pain clinics – a very useful liaison – as pain seems to be a major problem in management.
- Family involvement in terminal care is vital and most dying patients should be cared for in their own homes or hospices rather than acute medical wards.
- Patients vary with their threshold of pain – in some this may be disguised as aggression, confusion, debility and disturbed sleep.
- Pain may emanate from bony involvement or 'pressure' sores.

DEATHS IN BRONCHIAL CARCINOMA: WHAT FUTURE?

- Four out of five deaths in bronchial carcinoma are in men.

- Smoking is likely to remain a social problem – do lower tar content and filter tips of cigarettes have any part to play in lowering the risk involved? Evidence suggests that this is already happening[7]. Although in the male over 55 the mortality is rising, there is a fall in the under-45s. Female mortality (all ages) is rising.

- Air pollution has a part to play in aetiology: people in urban areas are 1.5 times more likely to develop the disease.

Therefore without a dramatic change in the attitudes of the public to the habit of smoking it is highly unlikely that deaths from lung cancer, of epidemic proportions now, will decrease in future.

References

1. Whimster, W. F. (1983). *Tumours of the Trachea, Bronchus, Lung and Pleura.* (London: Pitman)
2. Selawry, O. S. *et al.* (1977). Survival *Canc. Med.,* **39,** 1026–30
3. Higgins, G. A. *et al* (1975). *Arch. Surg.,* **110,** 570–5
4. Shields, T. W. *et al* (1972). *J. Thorac. Cardiovasc Surg.,* **64,** 391–9
5. McIntosh J. (1976). *Lancet,* **2,** 300
6. Aitken-Swan, J. (1959). *Br. Med. J.,* **1,** 779
7. Coggon, D. and Acheson, E. D. (1983). Trends in lung cancer mortality. *Thorax,* **38,** 722–3

8

Management of terminal illness

DEFINITION OF A TERMINAL ILLNESS

A terminal illness is generally regarded as being one from which the patient is not expected to recover. Cancer frequently causes terminal illness and may give rise to distressing symptoms. Non-malignant causes of terminal illness include

respiratory failure

cardiac failure

renal failure

neurological failure, e.g. motor neuron disease and multiple sclerosis

The management of malignant terminal illness can usually be applied to other terminal situations.

Good management of terminal illness starts with the diagnosis, usually first suspected clinically, and often later confirmed histologically.

Most patients are best managed with a simple honest explanation of their illness initially, especially when the eventual outcome is likely to be grave. Dishonesty on the part of the doctor at this stage may well jeopardize effective management later on.

WHO SHOULD MANAGE

The general practitioner is the key to good management of terminally ill patients.

He should be able to draw help from various specialties, whichever is appropriate during different stages of the illness.

The terminal care specialist nurse will often provide advice and help with the management. Her services will be invaluable and she will act as a link between the patient, his family, and the GP.

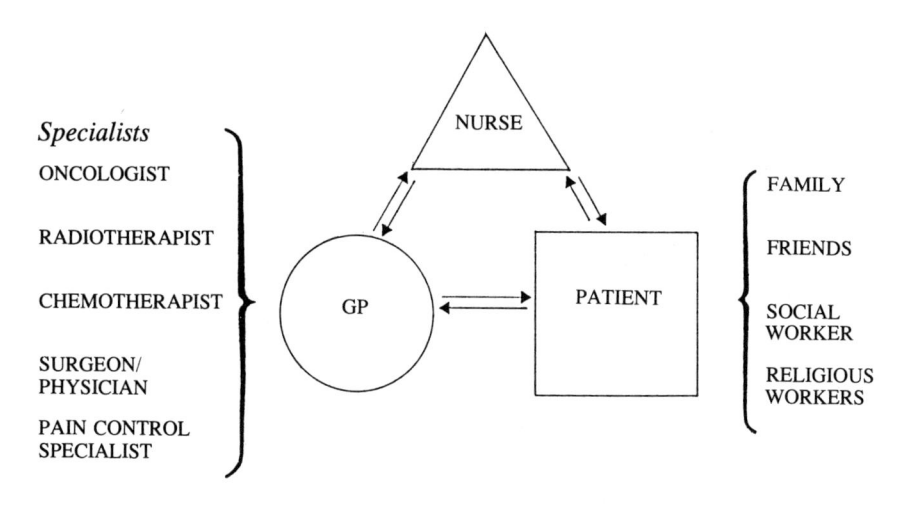

```
                            NURSE
                           /\
                          /  \
                         /    \
Specialists             /_____\
ONCOLOGIST             ↗        ↖
                      ↙          ↘              FAMILY
RADIOTHERAPIST    ┌─────┐    ┌─────────┐
                  │     │ →  │         │        FRIENDS
CHEMOTHERAPIST  → │ GP  │    │ PATIENT │
                  │     │ ←  │         │        SOCIAL
                  └─────┘    └─────────┘        WORKER
SURGEON/
PHYSICIAN                                       RELIGIOUS
                                                WORKERS
PAIN CONTROL
SPECIALIST
```

Many GPs prefer to manage their own terminally ill patients personally, placing themselves continuously on call. This represents a very great workload for the doctor but, of course, may be very satisfying.

If symptom control is difficult, and the illness prolonged, the patient may not be getting the best management. He might be better managed by a team of skilled terminal care nurses liaising closely with the GP.

WHERE TO MANAGE

A patient with terminal malignancy may be managed at home, in hospital or in a hospice unit, with sometimes combinations of all three at different stages of the illness.

Home management

In most cases home management will be ideal. The patient will be in familiar surroundings with friends and family in attendance. The GP plays the key role in managing his patient at home, drawing on specialist medical and nursing services as necessary and if available.

For successful home management, the following will be required.

(1) Suitable home conditions, with normal standards of accommodation, sanitation and access.
(2) Relatives or friends who are willing and able to look after the patient.
(3) Good symptom and nursing control.

Hospice management

A hospice unit will provide excellent care for a terminally ill patient. However, it may be some distance from the patient's home and family and this will mean difficulties in visiting the patient.

Hospital management

Hospital beds in Britain range from the acute medical and surgical beds in the District General Hospital to non-acute beds in the 'cottage hospitals', managed mainly by GPs.

A radiotherapy unit may well often manage dying patients, but this is not always the optimum use of beds and resources.

All hospital beds tend to be regimented, with fixed times for drug rounds, visiting and other hospital routines.

The terminally ill patient is not always best served by this routine although it may be necessary for the following reasons:

(1) overwhelming medical and nursing problems,
(2) no suitable home environment or relatives,
(3) no nearby hospice,
(4) patient's request to be in hospital, e.g. familiarity with surroundings and medical team.

The care of the terminally ill in acute hospitals is normally delegated to junior house staff, who often do not have the time, experience or interest in managing these patients. Similarly, senior medical and surgical staff tend to be more interested in saving life than improving the quality of life of those in whom death is inevitable.

Cottage hospital beds, usually managed by local GPs, offer the best environment for those in whom hospice or home management are not possible. The pace of life is slower, more relaxed and peaceful. There is good continuity of care from GPs who are often very skilled and experienced at dealing with the terminally ill.

HOW TO MANAGE THE TERMINALLY ILL

The object of good management is to diagnose and treat various unpleasant symptoms and signs, whether physical or emotional, as they arise, and on a continuing basis.

The diagnosis of terminal cancer is usually a devastating event, usually more so when the patient is young and has family and financial commitments. Good management will minimize or eliminate these feelings of devastation. Optimism on the part of the doctor, family and patient is usually worth while. In particular, the doctor must inspire confidence that unpleasant symptoms can be removed. By knowing there is a series of different treatments for a particular complaint, the patient may be reassured that if the first one does not satisfy, the next will be tried.

Most people associate cancer with a horrific demise, usually based on stories or experience of others who died with uncontrolled symptoms. A simple, honest explanation of the diagnosis, prognosis and unlikelihood of uncontrolled symptoms is required initially. Constant reassurance is needed during the progress of the illness so that feelings of hopelessness do not occur. Each new symptom should be investigated and dealt with promptly. Honesty about progress will almost always improve management.

UNPLEASANT SYMPTOMS OFTEN ASSOCIATED WITH MALIGNANCY

The most notable are

pain,
nausea and vomiting,
anxiety,
breathlessness,
confusion and restlessness and
constipation.

The management of pain in terminal illness

Not all patients with cancer experience pain. Not all admit true pain, preferring to call it stiffness or aching. Only after it has been relieved do they realize that it had been a form of pain.

Pain in cancer is due to the disease process in 75% of patients. In 20% of cancer patients with pain, it is probably secondary to treatment, particularly radiotherapy and chemotherapy, which are essentially destructive procedures. Inevitably nerve tissue is involved by these treatments and may give rise to unpleasant neuralgias or neuropathies which may be more troublesome for the patient than the disease itself.

The diagnosis of pain

This may be easy if there is an obvious expanding mass involving sensitive structures, or if X-rays or bone scans show secondary disease in appropriate areas such as the spine.

Quite often, examination and full investigation reveal no cause for pain. If a previous malignancy has occurred (even if many years ago) a clinical diagnosis may be made, based on the history and the time scale of the pain. In these cases, the pain is probably due to microscopic deposits of pain-producing neurotransmitters within the spinal cord. As yet, no test is available to establish the presence of these transmitters.

The causes of pain in malignancy

These are as follows:

(1) *Bone involvement*. Secondary deposits often produce prostaglandins and other pain-producing substances. Primary myelomatosis is usually painful for the same reason, and this is so specific that the pain level may be used to monitor the progress of the disease.

(2) *Nerve involvement*. Nerves may be compressed by tumour or infiltrated by tumour. Sudden compression may give sharp, shooting neuralgic pain followed by sensory and motor loss. Gradual compression will give gradual sensory and motor changes.

Infiltration of nerves by tumour may give burning dysaesthesiae in the appropriate area. There may also be hyperaesthesia. Sensory and motor changes usually follow.

(3) *Obstruction of ducts*, e.g. ureter, common bile duct, cervical canal, bowel, may produce a diffuse colicky pain with pain free intervals between attacks.

(4) *Direct tumour expansion* – with local invasion or sensitive structures or stretching of capsules, such as liver and kidney.

(5) *Infection, inflammation, necrosis* are usually potent causes of pain in malignancy, again due to production of potent pain-producing transmitters by the infective process.

Control of pain in terminal illness

Methods

These are

    pharmacological

surgical
radiotherapy
chemotherapy
nerve interruption

Pharmacological methods of pain control are usually quicker, more convenient and appropriate for the GP. They will be discussed in some detail.

Surgical relief of terminal pain implies surgical palliation of the malignancy where possible and appropriate.

Similarly radiotherapy and chemotherapy may relieve pain by palliating the underlying malignancy. Radiotherapy is usually effective in relieving pain from bony secondaries.

Nerve interruption will require the services of a specialist in this field. About 10% of all patients with terminal pain may benefit from a nerve block. This will be discussed later.

Drug control of pain

The analgesics may be divided into the following broad groups:

(1) Non-opioid analgesics
(2) Opioid analgesics
(3) Co-analgesics
    NSAIDs
    anxiolytics
    antidepressives
    anticonvulsants
    steroids

There are many regimens for the use of analgesic drugs. It is very important for the doctor to select as simple a regimen as possible, with the fewest tablets, using drugs that he is familiar with.

With the onset of pain in the earliest stages of the disease, a simple non-opioid analgesic may be started. Paracetamol, up to 1 g 4-hourly, is worth trying first. Soluble aspirin, up to 600 mg 4-hourly, or other variants to suit the patient, may work just as well.

From the moment this fails to give adequate analgesia, or the side-effects become troublesome, the addition of an opioid is necessary, particularly if the pain is becoming very severe. If the pain is almost controlled on a simple non-opioid, the addition of a co-analgesic may be worth trying before proceeding to an opioid.

Aqueous morphine 5–10 mg 4-hourly is a useful basic opioid to start with. It is simple, cheap, effective and very flexible in dosage, which is very useful at first. It may, however, induce nausea and constipation and therefore it is always important to add a prophylactic antiemetic and laxative, as opioid-induced nausea and constipation may become more troublesome than the pain. It may be possible to withdraw antiemetics later if nausea is not a problem.

Prochlorperazine tabs. 5 mg 4-hourly, with Dorbanex Forte 10 ml b.i.d. are useful prophylaxis.

Often commercial preparations of opioid plus non-opioid, such as Distalgesic, control early pain quite well, but not every patient is suited by this combination, and if the pain increases later, an increase in dose of this combined preparation may give undesirable side-effects.

Opioid antagonist analgesics (pentazocine, buprenorphine etc) may help with early pain but their usefulness is severely limited by a high incidence of side-effects, especially if the dose needs to be increased to control increased pain.

The patient should be warned that he or she may experience slight sedation when starting an opioid for the first time and again with each further dose increase. This sedation usually lasts only a few days, but always the incidence of side-effects must be balanced against the benefit from the drug.

When severe pain is the presenting symptom, urgent control is required. This means starting with a moderate dose of opioid and adjusting subsequent dose up or down, depending on the response to the previous dose.

Aqueous morphine is very flexible in dosage in the early stages of titration against the patient's pain. A suggested regimen is 10–20 mg orally, 4-hourly. A 4-hourly administration is best, because it approximates the useful length of action of oral aqueous morphine, and it is a reasonable time interval.

If pain is still present after the first 4 hours, the next dose should be 30 mg. If there is still pain at 4 hours, make another increase to 45 mg, then 60 mg, 90 mg, 120 mg and so on.

With higher doses, and when pain is controlled, the total 4-hourly dose should be made up in about 10 ml, as patients generally dislike larger volumes.

It is best to add nothing other than plain tap water to the morphine, as additives shorten the shelf life. Many patients dislike the taste of chloroform water, a common diluent and flavour, and some feel nauseated by the smell.

Morphine solution is bitter and this may be disguised by administration with another drink of the patient's choice, even tea or coffee.

When pain has been controlled in this way with aqueous morphine, a change may be made to a sustained action tablet such as MST Continus. Using the same 24 h dose, the equivalent dose of MST may be given, based on a twice-daily regimen.

The patient must be reviewed very frequently, as old pains disappear (allowing a reduction in analgesia) and new pains appear, requiring an increase or change in analgesic, or both.

The GP may well find the services of a community based hospice nursing service invaluable in managing these patients, particularly with the monitoring of their analgesia requirements. It is not always possible, necessary or appropriate for the GP to visit patients being managed in this way, every single day of their illness.

Co-analgesics

When pain control is not easily achieved using either a simple non-opiate or higher dose of opiate, the use of a co-analgesic must be considered.

There may be other symptoms such as vomiting and dyspnoea to deal with before total pain control can be achieved.

The *co-analgesic drug groups* are

non-steroidal anti-inflammatories (NSAIDs).
anxiolytics and tranquillizers
antidepressives
steroids
anticonvulsants
antibiotics

Non-steroidal anti-inflammatory drugs

These are most useful in controlling terminal pain, sometimes alone, but more often in combination with an opioid. 'Bone pain' will often require a NSAID for optimum control.

Flurbiprofen, up to 150 mg b.i.d. or naproxen 250–500 mg b.i.d. or suppository 500 mg b.i.d., are probably the optimum NSAIDs at the time of writing.

Indomethacin, although cheaper and very effective, has a higher incidence of unwanted side-effects.

Anxiolytics and tranquillizers

Anxiety is very often a prominent feature of a terminal illness. Good counselling and management of the illness is not always enough, and the addition of a small dose of an appropriate anxiolytic can transform a difficult situation.

Lorazepam, 1 mg t.i.d., is a useful anxiolytic in the benzodiazepine group, causing minimal sedation or other unwanted side-effects.

The phenothiazines have long been used as sedatives and analgesic potentiating drugs, in terminal illness. Although they are very useful as antiemetics or when profound sedation is required, they are not so useful if anxiety is the main problem. Their usefulness may be limited by anticholinergic side-effects such as dry mouth, constipation and blurred vision.

Antidepressives

Many patients on long-term opioids for pain control become depressed, but there is disagreement as to whether this is caused by the drug or the disease.

A trial of a tricyclic antidepressive is often worth while, starting with a low evening dose, increasing slowly over several days unless side-effects occur. If there is no improvement within a month, a change to another antidepressive may help, but if not they should be withdrawn.

Occasionally severe pain may only be controlled when an antidepressive is prescribed.

Amitryptiline 25 mg at night, increasing over a few days, is a useful antidepressive. Alternatives are the newer dothiepin 25 mg at night, or mianserin 20 mg at night or nomifensine 25–50 mg in the morning.

Steroids

These drugs are often of exceptional value in the control of malignant symptoms, such as pain, dyspnoea, vomiting, loss of appetite etc.

The more potent and convenient steroid dexamethasone tablets or injection may be used (potency ratio dexamethasone:prednisolone is 7:1).

Where the malignant pain is thought to be due to nerve compression or nerve infiltration by tumour, steroids are indicated, and good control of pain may only be possible with steroids, despite an already high dose of opioid. The following regimens are suggested:

(1) For improvement in appetite – dexamethasone tabs. 2 mg b.i.d.
(2) Nerve compression or infiltration pain – dexamethasone tabs. 4 mg b.i.d.
(3) Severe vomiting or headache, probably due to cerebral oedema – dexamethasone tabs. or inj. 8 mg b.i.d.

Higher doses of steroids (dexamethasone 16 mg a day, upwards) may be of use from time to time when symptoms are overwhelming and the patient's life expectancy is very short.

Indigestion, secondary to the use of steroids, occurs fairly often and it is important to control this promptly with simple antacids, mucosal protecting agents or the newer H_2-receptor antagonists such as cimetidine 200 mg b.i.d.

If there is no obvious clinical improvement after a week on steroids they should be withdrawn slowly at a suggested rate of 0.5 mg every 1–2 days.

Anticonvulsants

These are

> barbiturates
> carbamazepine
> phenytoin
> ethosuxamide
> sodium valproate
> benzodiazepines

Where pain is of a sharp, shooting, spasmodic nature, implying a neuralgic basis, an anticonvulsant may help.

Barbiturates are mildly antianalgesic and therefore not useful here.

Carbamazepine, phenytoin, ethosuxamide and sodium valproate are often limited by toxic side-effects and therefore not very useful.

In the benzodiazepine group, clonazepam has marked anticonvulsant activity and it is also analgesic when used in this way. It does not produce toxic side-effects although its usefulness may be limited by sedation, especially at first. A useful starting dose is 0.5 mg at night, increasing gradually to the point at which sedation becomes a problem.

Antibiotics

Infection often causes pain which may be poorly relieved by high doses of traditional analgesics. Antibiotics are always worth using in this situation, if they relieve pain. Even if infection is not clinically apparent, such as in oropharyngeal cancers without obvious ulceration, a trial of an appropriate antibiotic is worthwhile.

A simple broad-spectrum antibiotic such as amoxicillin may be tried first. If there is a likelihood of anaerobic infection (such as in oropharyngeal cancers or where there is surface ulceration) metronidazole should be added. The antibiotic should be withdrawn after a week or two if there is no clinical improvement in the pain by that time.

Where there is overwhelming infection causing severe pain and distress, the use of chloramphenicol should be considered, despite its toxicity in normal situations. Fungating necrotic tumours (e.g. breast), where there may be an offensive smell causing distress to the patient and family, should be treated in this way.

Control of nausea and vomiting in terminal illness

Although not so emotive as cancer pain, cancer-induced nausea and vomiting may in fact be just as troublesome, and even more difficult to control well.

Causes are

certain malignancies

bowel compression or obstruction by tumour

side-effects of opioid analgesics, chemotherapy or radiotherapy

raised intracranial pressure

Certain cancers, especially ovarian, cause marked nausea and vomiting, probably through an action on the chemoreceptor trigger zone, by circulating agents, as yet unidentified, produced by the tumour.

True bowel compression by tumour causing obstruction is fairly unusual. More likely the cause is profound constipation with ileus, secondary to the presence of tumour and opioid analgesia causing decreased bowel motility, inadequately prevented by laxatives and stool softeners.

The opioids frequently induce nausea, especially in females and when used for the first time. The patient may find this so unpleasant that further opioid analgesia is declined at any cost. It is thus better to prevent nausea than to try to treat it once it has occurred, and it may well be worth tolerating the side-effects of an effective antiemetic for the first few days.

The tendency to be nauseated usually diminishes with good control and prolonged illness. It does not necessarily increase with increased opioid dosage.

The management of nausea and vomiting relies initially on providing adequate blood levels of an appropriate antiemetic drug. Gastrointestinal bypass surgery is nearly always not indicated in these patients.

Oral administration of a simple antiemetic is usually adequate to prevent nausea, especially when starting an opioid for the first time. This relies on good drug absorption from the stomach or upper jejunum.

A suggested regimen is prochlorperazine tabs. 5 mg 4-hourly or suppositories 25 mg t.i.d.

If nausea does not develop after a week or two, the dose may be reduced or even stopped. Slight sedation may well occur at first and the patient should be warned to expect this.

Metoclopramide tabs. or syrup 10 mg 4-hourly may also prevent nausea and if not satisfactory on its own may be combined with prochlorperazine.

If nausea is worse on movement and activity, cyclizine 25–50 mg t.i.d. may be a more useful antiemetic, or it may be combined with metoclopramide or prochlorperazine.

If nausea is intractable on a simple regimen, the addition of haloperidol 1–2.5 mg b.i.d. may help, but extrapyramidal side-effects may be troublesome.

Where there is gastric stasis and vomiting, oral administration of antiemetics is inappropriate. Rectal or colostomal administration of prochlorperazine 25 mg t.i.d. may help. Analgesic suppositories may also be given in this way, as absorption is usually very reliable.

Traditional management of nausea and vomiting is 'nil by mouth', plus 'drip and suck' with a 4-hourly intramuscular antiemetic. This is not appropriate in the terminally ill.

Intramuscular injections of antiemetic may be required initially to obtain good control, but subsequent management should rely heavily on oral or rectal administration if possible.

Subcutaneous continuous infusions of antiemetics have recently become a practical possibility with the introduction of miniature portable battery-driven syringe pumps, which deliver a 24 h dose of antiemetic and analgesic. There is excellent absorption of drug and the smooth plasma drug profile gives good efficacy with minimal side-effects.

Where the above regimens have failed to control nausea and vomiting, steroids should be given, especially if there is associated loss of appetite, which is very common anyway in the later stages of terminal malignancy. Again, oral administration is to be preferred but, if this is not possible, betamethasone or dexamethasone 4–8 mg b.i.d. should be considered initially.

Control of breathlessness

Causes of breathlessness are

    major airway obstruction by tumour

    generalized small airway obstruction

    parenchymal damage due to tumour, DXT or chemotherapy causing fibrosis

    pulmonary oedema secondary to tumour

    pleural effusion

When there is dyspnoea in a terminal illness, the cause should be defined and removed if possible. Very often it is impossible to remove the cause, and management should then relieve the symptoms.

A simple bronchodilator salbutamol tabs. 2–4 mg t.i.d. or inhaler) may give marked symptomatic relief of breathlessness, even in the absence of clinical bronchospasm. Salbutamol 4–12 mg over 24 hours may also be given subcutaneously from a syringe driver.

The judicious use of opiates may improve breathlessness but at risk of worsening respiratory failure. A small dose should be given initially, such as aqueous morphine 5 mg 4-hourly, increasing very slowly over a few days to the point at which dyspnoea is relieved.

When there is severe breathlessness and the patient is too weak to talk or eat, opioids may relieve distress very effectively for the first day or two before precipitating respiratory failure. The family and patient (if appropriate) should be warned of this possibility.

Steroids may relieve malignant breathlessness very effectively, despite their tendency to cause fluid retention. They should not be withheld for this reason even in the presence of peripheral oedema.

Pleural drainage may give good relief of breathlessness where an effusion is present. The relief obtained from a single drainage procedure may last for days or weeks, although there is a small risk of causing a permanently draining pleural fistula, but this is not usually troublesome.

Oxygen therapy is physiologically inappropriate in patients with terminal breathlessness although the presence of an oxygen cylinder by the patient's bed has a marked placebo effect. Also, the inhalation of cool dry gas may have a mild bronchodilating effect thus giving a sensation of relief of breathlessness.

If there is severe anxiety associated with breathlessness, simple relaxation, modified yoga or antenatal breathing exercises may help.

Superior vena cava obstruction

Continuous subcutaneous frusemide 150 mg over 24 hours using a syringe driver may help, although urinary catheterization is advisable.

Control of other unpleasant symptoms

Dry mouth

A dry mouth is usually secondary to drug treatment, disease or fungal infection, and it may be most unpleasant for the patient. An artificial saliva spray may help, such as Glandosane. Glandosane is now available on prescription from Dylade Ltd, 45 Brindley Road, Astmoore Industrial Estate, Runcorn WA7 1PG; tel. Runcorn 65011.

Sore mouth

This is usually due to oral candidiasis and therefore best treated with an antifungal such as nystatin suspension 1 ml q.i.d. or the newer ketoconazole tabs. 200 mg b.i.d.

Night sweats

Cause unknown, but they are a fairly common complaint in those with terminal malignancy. Indomethacin is sometimes effective.

THE MANAGEMENT OF CATASTROPHES IN TERMINAL ILLNESS

Where death is inevitable from a malignancy, many patients fear an unpleasant catastrophic end, especially if their malignancy happens to be situated in the mouth, throat, neck or chest.

Fears include:

choking or suffocating to death

bleeding to death from haemoptysis or haematemesis

general disintegration of body, such as in burst abdomen, or when there is a fungating necrotic tumour on the body surface

Patients should be very strongly reassured that these forms of death are most unlikely.

True respiratory obstruction due to tumour, causing death from suffocation, is rare. If obstruction seems a possibility, high dose steroids or radiotherapy, if possible, should be given to reduce local obstruction, buying time so that the malignant process eventually causes the patient's death in a more peaceful and less dramatic way.

Massive haemoptysis or haematemesis do occur from time to time and may be the actual cause of death, especially if the malignancy is pulmonary or gastric.

When death from this cause appears inevitable, the use of intravenous opioids plus sedation is appropriate. The slow i.v. injection of diamorphine 5–10 mg will relieve pain and start to relieve distress.

Hyoscine 0.6–2.4 mg i.v. or i.m. will exert a marked calming effect on the patient even while he or she is exsanguinating.

If vomiting and choking are happening at the same time, hyoscine will minimize these reflexes, and should the patient happen to recover from this unfortunate episode there may be a degree of amnesia from the hyoscine.

Traditionally, large doses of a heavy sedative such as chlorpromazine are reserved for such emergencies, but the quality of relief with hyoscine is much higher than that with chlorpromazine.

PHYSICAL AIDS TO THE MANAGEMENT OF THE TERMINALLY ILL

Flowtron

This is a pneumatic intermittent compression device for the relief of symptoms of lymphoedema in a limb. It often gives excellent symptomatic relief in secondary lymphoedema in the arm from axillary malignancy from cancer of the breast.

Ozonette

This is an electrical device for minimizing offensive smells from necrotic, fungating tumours.

Ripple mattresses

These minimize the occurrence of painful pressure sores in the bedbound.

Wheelchairs

Wheelchairs and other aids to mobility may be required at fairly short notice, obtained usually from the community nursing services. The Red Cross organization in some areas may also be able to provide wheelchairs for short-term use. Long-term wheelchairs are obtained usually from the regional limb fitting centre but may take up to 3 months after ordering, which is not appropriate in terminal patients.

Rearrangement of accommodation

Moving the patient's bed downstairs or next door to the bathroom is often a simple practical exercise which helps management. A telephone extension improves communication, and most local telephone offices will be sympathetic to the installation of a new telephone line as a matter of urgency.

ENTONOX ANALGESIA

Premixed cylinders of nitrous oxide and oxygen in a 50 : 50 ratio (entonox) are most useful for providing high quality short-term analgesia for painful or stimulating procedures such as changing of dressings or packs.

A fungating discharging tumour that needs frequent dressing changes will often be very sensitive. Large doses of opioids and other analgesics beforehand rarely provide enough analgesia to allow the dressings to be changed. By administration of analgesics in this way, the patient is subjected to several hours' worth of extra analgesia with probable sedation which he does not require.

The onset and duration of entonox is extremely short (a few minutes) and as there is no accumulation of drug, there are no after-effects.

Midwives are legally permitted to administer entonox to patients in their own right. In the care of terminal patients, nursing staff without a midwifery qualification should also be able to administer entonox to patients, following instruction from a doctor and certification by local nursing and medical administration.

CONTINUOUS SUBCUTANEOUS INFUSIONS

Continuous subcutaneous infusions of analgesics, antiemetics and other drugs are now a practical possibility with the availability of miniature, battery-operated syringe pumps. As the rate of injection is very slow, subcutaneous administration of most drugs results in perfectly adequate plasma drug levels.

Indications are

(1) patient unable to swallow medication (too ill or too sick)

(2) oral analgesics or antimetics not effective enough

(3) good control of distress occurring within a day or two of death

Drugs may be given singly or mixed in the same syringe and given over 24 hours. Although this is pharmacologically undesirable, in practice it works extremely well.

Diamorphine is the analgesic of choice, owing to its high solubility, potency and good absorption. Half the current total daily oral intake is a useful starting dose. There is plenty of time to monitor the effects of a subcutaneous infusion, so that the dose may be modified if necessary after several hours.

Metoclopramide mixes well with diamorphine although the resulting solution is of high volume, which may restrict the addition of other drugs in the same syringe.

Haloperidol 2.5–5 mg over 24 hours is a useful additional antiemetic if metoclopramide is insufficient on its own.

The phenothiazines, however, although appearing to be chemically compatible in the same syringe, tend to cause increased skin reactions at the site of injection and should probably not be given in this way.

The exception among phenothiazines is methotrimeprazine (Nozinan, Veractil). This powerful phenothiazine may potentiate analgesia and is also a powerful antiemetic. Dose range is 25–150 mg over 24 hours.

Steroids are not compatible with analgesics being given in this way. They are, however, very soluble and easily absorbed when administered in other ways.

Solutions are administered subcutaneously using a 21g 'Butterfly' needle inserted over the abdominal wall if the patient is in bed, or over the scapula if he is mobile. The 'Butterfly' needle is connected to the syringe by 0.6 M fine bore plastic tubing and the site of insertion is best inspected daily and changed from time to time as necessary.

THE PLACE OF NERVE BLOCKS IN MALIGNANT PAIN

Probably 10% of all patients dying from a malignancy could be helped in some way from a nerve block. Nerves may be blocked as follows:

(1) local anaesthetic

(2) chemical destruction with alcohol, phenol or chlorocresol

(3) freezing destruction (cryoprobe)

(4) thermocoagulation (radio frequency lesion generator)

Local anaesthetic nerve blocks are usually worth trying initially as the relief of pain may outlast the known duration of block. The mechanism for this apparent action is unknown. Local anaesthetic blocks are generally very safe and may give the patient an indication of what to expect if a permanent block is carried out.

Indications for a nerve block

These are

(1) rapidly escalating doses of analgesia without corresponding improvement

(2) unacceptable side-effects from current analgesic regime

(3) patient's dislike of taking drugs

(4) localized pain breaking through otherwise adequate analgesia

For a nerve block to be acceptable in the management, access to suitable facilities and specialist should be possible.

Useful nerve blocks

Coeliac plexus sympathetic block

Usually with absolute alcohol up to 20 ml anterior to the body of L1, best performed with X-ray image intensification, but may be performed 'blind' if the patient is too ill to move.

Often good relief of abdominal visceral pain, such as from carcinoma of the head of the pancreas, and may help to control vomiting from the same cause.

Epidural injection of local anaesthetic and steroid

Quite good relief from this block in patients with spinal metastases, with relief outlasting known short duration of local anaesthetic.

Intrathecal nerve root blocks

Fairly good results in experienced hands for pain localized to the lower half of the body, especially if unilateral. There is a marked risk to bladder function with lumbosacral neurolytic blocks.

Thoracic paravertebral nerve blocks

May be useful for unilateral rib or girdle pain.

Interscalene brachial plexus blocks

May be useful where there is intractable pain in the arm, usually from carcinoma of the breast with local secondary disease. Patients should have a trial block with local anaesthetic, as the numbness produced may be more unpleasant than the pain.

Local anaesthetic injection of painful trigger points

Tender muscular trigger points may occur from time to time in terminal malignancy. Their explanation is unknown at present. Pain elsewhere may otherwise be well controlled, and a painful trigger point may then become a problem.

Injection of the point with 5–10 ml of plain local anaesthetic often results in relief of pain, frequently permanently, or if not permanent, much improved.

FINANCIAL HELP FOR THE TERMINALLY ILL

Financial help in the form of allowances and grants may be possible in certain circumstances.

Contributory invalidity pension

This is automatic after 26 weeks' illness if claiming sickness benefit.

Non-contributory invalidity pension (NI 210)

This is available for people of working age who have not been able to work for 6 months and cannot get sickness or invalidity benefit because they have not paid enough National Insurance contributions. It is tax-free and not means-tested.

Non-contributory invalidity pension for married women (NI 214)

This is available for married women who have not been able to work for 6 months, and do not qualify for sickness and invadility benefit because they have not paid enough National Insurance contributions. It is also available to married women who are both incapable of doing paid work and incapable of carrying out normal household duties. In the latter situation the benefit is referred to as HCNIP. It is tax-free and not means-tested.

This benefit is due to become *the severe disability allowance*, and will only be granted to housewives with an 80% disability.

Supplementary benefit (Pension)

An extra food and heating allowance is paid following an explanatory letter from the doctor (GP or consultant).

Attendance allowance (NI 205)

This is available in cases of severe disability for 6 months requiring frequent attention throughout the 24 h period, in connection with bodily function. Or when continual supervision is required to prevent damage to the patient or others.

Mobility allowance (NI 211)

This is payable to those who have a physical condition which renders them incapable, or virtually incapable, of walking, or the exertion to walk is life-threatening. The condition must be likely to last for 1 year and the patient must be able to make use of the allowance (i.e. must not be comatose).

Prescription exemption (FP 91)

This is available to those who have a permanent physical disability which prevents them leaving their residence, except with the help of another person. It is automatically available to those receiving Supplementary Benefit or Family Income Supplement, and those suffering from certain benign chronic illnesses.

Domiciliary visits by dentists and opticians

These are free to those on supplementary benefit or pension.

The British Dental Association (01-935 0875) will provide the name of a suitable local dentist if the patient's own dentist is unable to visit.

The National Society for Cancer Refief

The Society may be able to provide grants in certain circumstances, and following a report from a doctor.

Special grants may be made for the following:

a large heating bill
installation of a telephone
a holiday
mortgage arrears
hospital visiting expenses

9

Tuberculosis

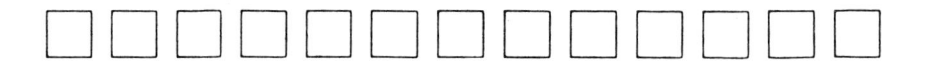

☐ ☐ ☐ ☐ ☐ ☐ ☐ ☐ ☐ ☐ ☐ ☐

SIGNIFICANCE

- In terms of total annual notifications (15 000), still a relatively common problem.
- Ranks as one of 'top six' causes of weight loss in United Kingdom.
- There are 30 000 general practitioners in the UK, therefore less than one new case every 2 years, whilst a consultant in a 'high risk' area may see one to two new cases per month.
- May present in 'unusual' fashion (*see below*).
- Need for strict vigilance in vulnerable groups.
- Asian, male, middle-aged immigrants at a special risk (as no primary immunity and 'change' in immune state at middle age).
- Future trends for TB unpredictable.
- Mortality in newly notified cases (England and Wales) is still significant. Analysing 1312 adult patients[1] of white and Indian origin – with pulmonary disease only – over a 6-month period:

  > 163 (12%) died before completing treatment.
  >   96% were white
  >   1:2 deaths as direct result of pulmonary TB

- Those who died, 70% did so over the first 4 weeks of treatment.
- In 51 adults, out of the total of 1312, the diagnosis was made after death.

TB deaths (at risk)
- Old (not related to sex of patient)
- Extensive cavitating disease (on chest X-ray)
- Smear positive

Common causes of weight loss in UK, 6 kg × 6 weeks
- Carcinoma
- Diabetes mellitus
- *Tuberculosis*
- Thyrotoxicosis
- Depression/anorexia nervosa
- Malabsorption and inflammatory bowel disease

Patients vulnerable to tuberculosis
- Alcoholics
- Male Asians (middle aged) (500:100 000 as compared to 7:100 000 native white population)
- Diabetics
- Immunosuppressed
- Those with chronic lung disorders (anonymous mycobacterium infections)
- Previous peptic ulcer surgery
- Related to occupation: *silicosis; Caplan's*
- Previous disease (inadequate, inappropriate or insufficient treatment)

Organisms causing tuberculosis:
(acid fast bacilli)

Mycobacterium tuberculosis
- Human
- Bovine (non-pasteurized milk – abdominal disease)
- Avian
- Murine

Anonymous (atypical)
(OPPORTUNISTIC INFECTION)
- *Mycobacterium intracellularae*
- *Mycobacterium kansasii*
- *Mycobacterium xenopi*

Anonymous mycobacterium infection: features

- Diagnosis can only be made following repeated (up to nine) positive sputum results
- Patient will be aged 50 and over
- May complicate pneumoconiosis
- On the whole, clinical features as for other mycobacterium infection
- Lymph nodes likely to be enlarged

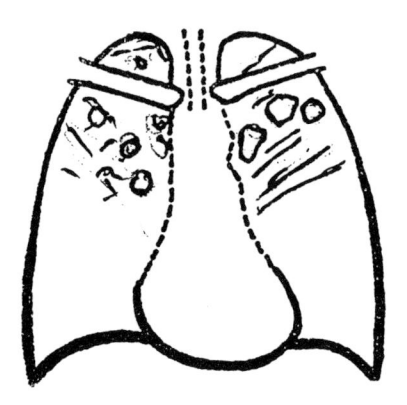

- Multiple (four or five) drug combinations necessary. Culture/sensitivity of sputum to guide. Problem in drug compliance. Hospital supervision of therapy necessary

CLINICAL TYPES

- Primary tuberculosis
- Postprimary tuberculosis
- Miliary disease
- Pneumonic infiltration
- Pleural tuberculosis
- Anonymous mycobacterium disease

TUBERCULOSIS

Primary tuberculosis

- Type of patient
  - Immigrants and children under the age of 11 who are contacts of cases of active TB. Occasionally in elderly patients
- Symptoms
  - Often asymptomatic. Dry cough, fever and constitutional symptoms may exist. ? Erythema nodosum
- Chest X-ray
  - May be confused with sarcoidosis, Hodgkin's and carcinoma

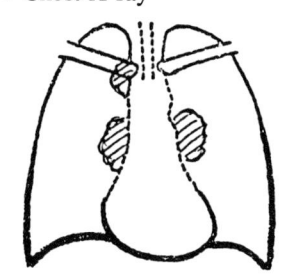

Hilar and paratracheal nodes

Post-primary tuberculosis

- Type of patient
  - Usually indigenous, middle-aged – possibly alcoholics. May have a previous history of TB
- Symptoms
  - Cough, sputum, haemoptysis, night sweats, weight loss
- Chest X-ray
  - May be confused with old sarcoid, aspergillosis, allergic alveolitis and ankylosing spondylitis

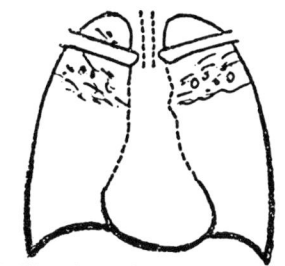

Infiltration of upper zones. Cavitation/reticulation

Miliary tuberculosis

- Type of patient
  - The very young (under 10 years) and very old (over 75 years). Many diagnosed at postmortem. Also possible in immunosuppressed

- Symptoms
  - May be asymptomatic. Weight loss and constitutional upset. May present as tuberculosis meningitis (TBM)

- Chest X-ray
  - Radiological features are usually specific but unusual infections and reticulo-endothelial disease, e.g. Hodgkin's, can give similar appearances

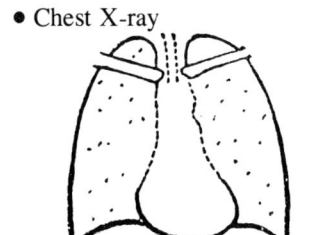

Punctate/nodular
– occasionally calcified lesions on both lung fields

Pneumonic infiltration

- Type of patient
  - Rare
- Symptoms
  - Can present as a severe pneumonic illness with breathlessness, cough and haemoptysis, chest pain (pleuritic)

- Chest X-ray
  - Differential diagnosis of atypical pneumonia (*see below*). Mainly apical or posterior segment of the upper lobes

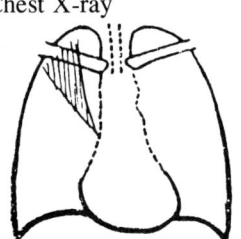

Could be segmental or lobar. May cavitate

Pleural tuberculosis

- Type of patient
  - A previous small focus of infection within lung causes hypersensitive reaction on the pleura
- Symptoms
  - Breathlessness, pain (pleuritic) and weight loss
- Chest X-ray
  - Differential diagnosis of pleural effusion especially pneumonia, cancer

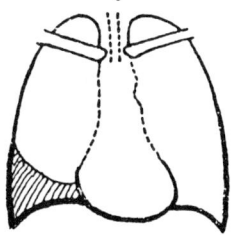

Usually unilateral. Occasionally bilateral large effusion

Anonymous mycobacterium

- Type of patient
  - Those with longstanding infiltrative/destructive lung disorders. Can especially complicate lung fibrosis, aspergillosis and progressive massive fibrosis (PMF)
- Symptoms
  - Breathlessness, weight loss, haemoptysis. Repeated (6–9) positive sputa results necessary
- Chest X-ray
  - Differential diagnosis of upper lobe fibrosis

Usually apical (bilateral) upper zone shadowing

UNUSUAL CLINICAL PRESENTATIONS OF TUBERCULOSIS

- Confusion
- Arthritis

- Skin lesions and erythema nodosum (primary TB)

- Pott's disease

- Haematuria

- Ascites

- May suggest tuberculous meningitis
- Effusion usually symmetrical. Bony involvement will lead to osteomyelitis
- Erythema induratum (Bazin's disease) will present as ulcerating chilblain-like lesions over the calves of the legs. Lupus vulgaris – destructive nasal lesion
- Now rare – paravertebral cold abscess
- Often painless, suggesting renal tract TB
- May present with acute abdomen (bovine form of TB)

TUBERCULOSIS

Conditions which may mimic tuberculosis (human)

- Anonymous mycobacterial infections

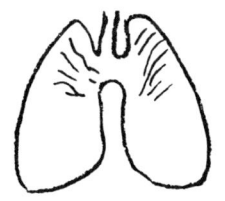

- Granulomatous disorders

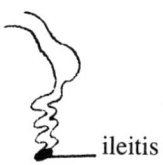

  — in the gastrointestinal tract, e.g. Crohn's disease
  — ileitis

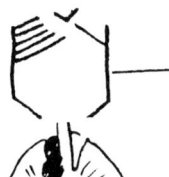

  — in the liver, e.g. non-specific granulomatosis conditions

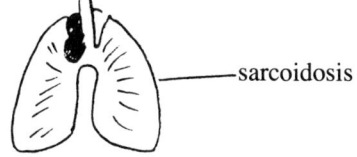

  — sarcoidosis

- Lymphadenopathy due to reticuloses

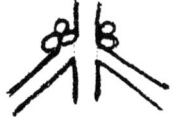

- Meningitis (lymphocytic)

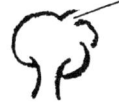

- Peritonitis ('bovine' TB)

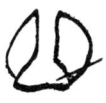

- Heart disease
  — pericardial effusion
  — cardiomyopathy

DIAGNOSIS

> *Diagnosis of tuberculosis*
>
> - HISTOLOGY
>   Biopsy of a lymph node
>   Curettage (gynaecological procedures)
>   Scalene node
> - MICROBIOLOGY
>   Three specimens of sputa for Ziehl–Nielsen staining and Löwenstein culture
>   Three early morning urine specimens (EMU)
>   Fluid obtained from abscess, cerebrospinal space and stomach
>   Nasal, throat, pharyngeal swabs
> - TUBERCULIN TESTING
>   Measure induration at 36 and 72 hours, a positive result is >5 mm
> - FUNDOSCOPY
>   Choroid tubercles

PROBLEMS

- In spite of strong clinical suspicion, the microbiology and histology may return negative.
- Tuberculin test may fail to give a positive result in
    disseminated or miliary TB
    concurrent Hodgkin's, carcinoma and sarcoid
    immunosuppressive and steroid therapy
    poor technique
    ineffective tuberculin reagent
- Cases of bovine tuberculosis may not present with 'lung features' and could be mistaken in the gut as Crohn's disease.
- When delay in diagnosis, the disease will disseminate and carries a significant mortality.
- Extensive lung involvement may produce pneumothoraces, fibrosis, bronchiectasis, recurrent haemoptysis and aspergillosis. These patients will eventually become 'respiratory cripples'.
- Patients who had in the past undergone thoracoplasty, phrenic crush, artificial pneumothorax and pneumoperitoneum are still seen with significant restrictive lung disorder.
- Effects of discontinuing BCG vaccination and facilities for routine chest X-rays are unpredictable. It is possible that yearly notification may rise.

TUBERCULOSIS

- Future of contact-tracing?

Management

- Isolation is not always necessary.
- Fifty per cent of diagnosed cases could be treated at home. These include:
  (1) those with no cough, sputum, sneezing or discharging wound
  (2) those with extrapulmonary TB with consistent negative sputa results
  (3) patient with good 'social' support – relatives who may supervise therapy
- Those treated in hospital:
  (1) alcoholics
  (2) drug resistant infection
  (3) with other concurrent disorders
  (4) poor living standards
  (5) extensive 'open' disease
- It is now agreed that 6–9 months chemotherapy is sufficient for all forms of mycobacterium tuberculosis. 'Anonymous' infection and extrapulmonary disease will need therapy for up to 18 months. The simple principle of continuing therapy for long enough period to eradicate the disease is a good one.
- Apart from drugs, withdrawal of alcohol, rest and a good diet is necessary.
- Resistance to commonly used antituberculosis drugs, especially isoniazid, is becoming more significant.
- Regular visits by practice nurse/health visitor to supervise therapy should be encouraged.
- Regular follow-up at doctor's surgery to discuss difficulties in therapy.

Contact tracing[2]

- Still most useful way of controlling TB in a community
- All cases of pulmonary and extrapulmonary disease must be notified – a GP has responsibility to make sure that they are
- Children under 13 years skin tested; if tuberculin/Heaf positive – a chest X-ray may be necessary. The Tine test is convenient but not reliable. BCG offered to Heaf grade 0–1 contacts unless they have been vaccinated before
- Chemoprophylaxis (isoniazid) offered to strongly positive reactors
- Chest X-ray necessary for adults. They should be referred to Chest Clinic for follow-up

DRUG THERAPY

Most commonly used combination:

rifampicin } also available as Rimactizid '150'; Rifinah '300'
isoniazid }
ethambutol } also available as Mynah '400'; Myambutol

Other drugs available:

streptomycin
pyrazinamide
thiacetazone
para-amino salicylic acid (PAS)
capreomycin
ethionamide

Favoured regimen

For first 2 months, triple therapy:

rifampicin } as Rifinah, Rimactizid '150', '300'
isoniazid }
ethambutol } as Mynah, Myambutol

After this period:

(1) omit ethambutol (if 'badly' tolerated, renal or eye involvement)

(2) or omit rifampicin (if jaundice, anorexia, diarrhoea)

(3) and continue Rifinah or Mynah for 6–12 months

    (a) regular sputa for *sensitivity*
    (b) *adjust therapy* accordingly

TUBERCULOSIS

• *Rifampicin* (in children: 12 mg/kg b.w.) In adults > 50 kg b.w.: 600 mg/day. < 50 kg b.w.: 450 mg/day	• Highly effective • Bactericidal • Nausea, vomiting • Discolours urine, saliva, sweat and tears (orange-pink) • Abnormalities of liver function (transaminases) *alcoholics • Precaution with the *contraceptive pill *antiepileptics, esp. phenytoin *anticoagulants • Avoid in pregnancy • Marrow dysfunction and bruising is rare • Can be detected in the urine – a help in assessing compliance
• *Isoniazid* In children 5 mg/kg b.w. In adults 200–300 mg/day	• Effective • Bactericidal • Fever, rash • At high dose – pyridoxine 10 mg/day to avoid peripheral neuropathy • Hepatotoxicity rare
• *Ethambutol* Safe dose – 15 mg/kg b.w. Larger dose – 25 mg/kg b.w.	• Effective – not well tolerated • Bacteriostatic, therefore a useful combination with isoniazid or rifampicin • Ophthalmological check especially with larger dose and previous history of eye diseases *may produce optic neuritis *disturbance of visual acuity and colour vision • Avoid in children, very old and those with poor renal function.

• *Streptomycin* < 40 years 1 g/day > 40 years 0.5–0.75 g/day	• Injections only – a disadvantage but useful in supervised therapy causes vestibular toxicity hypersensitive reactions occur nephrotoxic rarely hirsutism

• *Pyrazinamide*
    >50 kg 2 g/day
    <50 kg 1.5 g/day
    (single dose)
	• Bactericidal
	• Poorly tolerated
	• Hepatitis, photosensitivity, hyperuricaemia and arthralgia
	• Specially useful in TBM

• *Thiacetazone*	• Rarely used in UK • May be effective in anonymous mycobacterium
• *PAS*	• Useful in children, poorly tolerated by adults • Nausea, vomiting, diarrhoea • Goitre and hypothyroidism rare
• *Capreomycin*	• Useful in TB resistant to first-line drugs • Side-effects common
• *Cycloserine*	• Neurological and renal side-effects

Corticosteroids in tuberculosis
(Prednisone 30 mg/day)

- In very ill patients with disseminated disease
- When the pleura, eyes and pericardium are involved
- Indicated in some cases of TBM
- Very useful in treating hypersensitivity reactions
- In Addison's disease (hypoadrenalism), cortisone is preferred to prednisone

> ### *Hypersensitivity to antituberculosis drugs*
> - Could cause a serious problem
> - Identify the drug causing hypersensitivity
> - Try to avoid that drug
> - If choice limited, use steroids

References
1. Humphries, M. J. *et al.* (1984). *Br. J. Dis. Chest,* **78,** 149
2. Control and prevention of T.B. – a code of practice. (1983). *Br. Med. J.*, **287,** 1083–1156

10

Sarcoidosis

SIGNIFICANCE

- A granulomatous disorder.
- Is being increasingly recognized.
- The majority do not need any specific treatment.
- Significance of the diagnosis should be explained to the patient.
- Extrapulmonary disease may take unpredictable and protracted course and need careful assessment and follow-up.
- Most GPs would see two or three cases during lifetime. Some geographical variation. Commoner amongst the Irish and West Indians.

Clinical types

Useful to classify pulmonary sarcoidosis in the radiological groups:

SARCOIDOSIS

Unilateral/bilateral hilar lymphadenopathy (BHL)
± paratracheal node

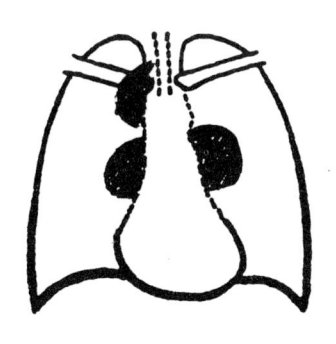

Can be mistaken for primary tuberculosis especially in an immigrant

Erythema nodosum often present (red nodules over the front of legs and extensor aspects of arms)

Females > males (aged 25–40)

Constitutional symptoms may occur

- fever
- arthralgia
- malaise

Most (95%) clear spontaneously

Erythema nodosum and sarcoidosis (EN)

May coincide with, precede or follow the finding of bilateral hilar glandular enlargement (BHL)

Red, slightly painful lesions in 'crops'

Other causes, e.g. the birth-control 'pill', antibiotics (penicillin and sulphonamides), tuberculosis, leprosy

The association of EN + BHL is sometimes called *Loffgren's* syndrome and 20% of patients with sarcoidosis will present with this combination

Reticulocavitating disease

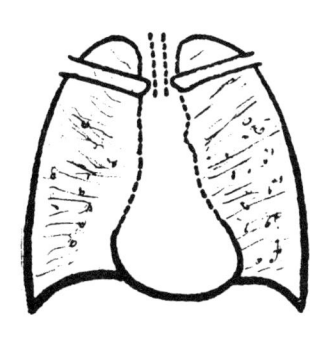

- Wide differential diagnosis (infiltrative lung disorders) – *see below*
- Affects mainly mid and upper zones of the lungs
- May complicate (BHL)
- Erythema nodosum rare
- Older patient – especially Irish and West Indian
- Present with breathlessness
- Need detailed assessment

> *Differential diagnosis of diffuse pulmonary infiltrate*
>
> Sarcoidosis
> Tuberculosis
> Lymphoma
> Lymphangitis carcinomatosis
> Extrinsic and fibrosing alveolitis
> Pulmonary aspergillosis and eosinophillia
> Collagen disorders
> Pneumoconiosis, berylliosis
> Histoplasmosis
> Infections especially 'viral'
> Drug reactions

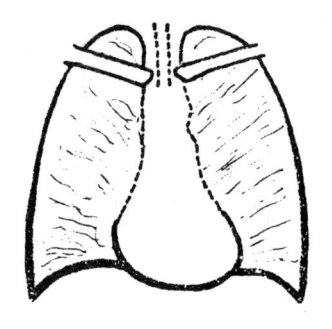

PROBLEMS

Those diagnosed on routine chest X-rays and found to have BHL and erythema nodosum (EN) should be reassured. A further film necessary in 12 months, or earlier if new symptoms appear (chronic cough and breathlessness). Unless suggestion of other extrapulmonary features, referral to hospital not necessary.

Histological evidence is required in patients in whom the diagnosis is not certain and those presenting with reticulocavitating lung disease and extrapulmonary disorders.

A positive Kveim/Siltzbach test is finding on histology of non-caseating epitheliod granulomas. Positive result in only two thirds of cases. False positives in 2% of patients with variety of other disorders.

Elevated levels of serum angiotensin converting enzyme known to occur in about 60% of patients. Many cases of interstitial lung disease will give a positive result.

Pulmonary function tests normal in the common form of sarcoidosis with BHL. In infiltrative disease, a restrictive pattern FEV_1/FVC reduced equally but ratio $\approx 80\text{--}85\%$. Transfer factor of carbon monoxide (TCO) markedly reduced.

Hypercalcaemia > 2.8 mmol/l occurs in 10% of cases only. Phosphate is normal or slightly increased. IgE levels raised in some cases.

SARCOIDOSIS

Extrapulmonary manifestations

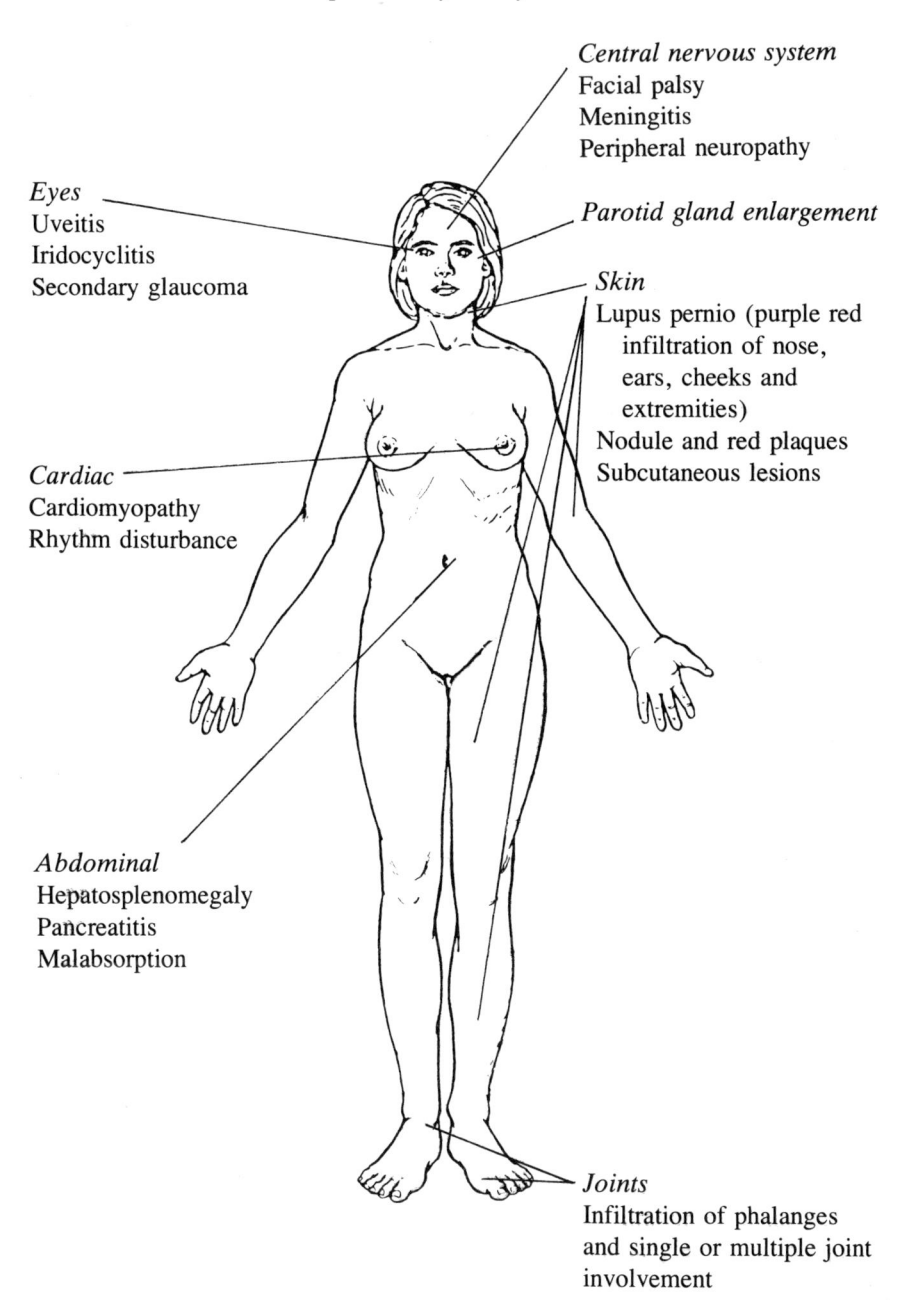

Central nervous system
Facial palsy
Meningitis
Peripheral neuropathy

Eyes
Uveitis
Iridocyclitis
Secondary glaucoma

Parotid gland enlargement

Skin
Lupus pernio (purple red infiltration of nose, ears, cheeks and extremities)
Nodule and red plaques
Subcutaneous lesions

Cardiac
Cardiomyopathy
Rhythm disturbance

Abdominal
Hepatosplenomegaly
Pancreatitis
Malabsorption

Joints
Infiltration of phalanges and single or multiple joint involvement

COURSE AND DRUG MANAGEMENT

The vast majority of patients with sarcoidosis can expect a benign course, with complete clearing or non-disabling persistence of radiographic and other clinical abnormalities.

A significant proportion (although small) will be disabled probably temporarily.

Four per cent develop respiratory failure and die. Sarcoid cardiomyopathy, renal failure, aspergilloma and sarcoid bullae may also kill.

Only 10% of patients with deteriorating pulmonary function tests will need long-term mandatory steroids.

Drugs used

STEROIDS

CHLOROQUINE

? OTHER IMMUNOSUPPRESSIVES

INDOMETHACIN
(and other prostaglandin inhibitors)

Corticosteroids and sarcoidosis

Active sarcoidosis responds well to corticosteroids.

Discussions on the dose and duration.

Relatively small dose will shrink a granuloma.

Practice to continue therapy for 6–9 months.

Cessation of therapy may cause relapse especially in cutaneous sarcoidosis. In these chloroquine-trial may be justified. (N.B. ophthalmological complications of chloroquine.)

Steroids and sarcoidosis

Prompt, mandatory treatment (collaboration with a specialist) in

Central nervous involvement

Eye involvement (ophthalmological opinion necessary)

Hypercalcaemia

Cardiomyopathy

A few cases of interstitial lung disease

Therapy necessary in 20%

Persistent constitutional symptoms

Large painful salivary glands and lymph node

Upper airways mucosal lesions

Peripheral neuromuscular disorders

Steroids not indicated in

Asymptomatic hilar lymphadenopathy

Minor radiographic abnormality

Erythema nodosum will respond to indomethacin (25 mg t.d.s. for 2–3 weeks only), aspirin

---

Dose of steroids

Initial dose of prednisone 45 mg/day reduced over 6–8 weeks to 10 mg/day. No advantage in alternate day regime. Enteric-coated preparation preferred in those with dyspepsia and previous history of peptic ulcer.

Short duration 6–9 months in

(1) hypercalcaemia,
(2) symptoms of acute sarcoidosis.

Longer duration $\approx$ 2 years in

chronic progressive pulmonary/extrapulmonary disease.

11

Acute infections of the lungs

SIGNIFICANCE

- Frequent – potentially dangerous
  mortality 200 : 100 000 population
- Probably most serious conditions treated by a general practitioner
- Special risk to
  infants
  'chronic chests'
  immunosuppressed
  those with other medical conditions, e.g. diabetes mellitus, renal failure and cardiac disease
- Effective therapy possible in most of the cases
- Need for careful supervision, investigations and follow-up

WHAT ARE THEY?

- The pneumonias
- Acute bronchitis
- Pleurisy
- Infected infarction and septic emboli
- Lung abscess

ACUTE INFECTIONS OF THE LUNGS

Causative organisms (common)	
Bacterial	*Viral and 'others'*
Streptococcus pneumoniae	influenza virus
Haemophilus influenzae	RSV virus
Streptococcus pyogenes	Mycoplasma

THE PNEUMONIAS

Aetiology

- *Following severe upper respiratory tract infection.*
- Chronic infection (bronchitis/bronchiectasis) may cause *infected material* to be aspirated especially *from sinuses.*
- Certain types of *hiatus hernia* and *achalasia* may cause aspiration of contents into the lungs especially when the patient is in bed.
- Regular use of *paraffin* in the elderly may cause recurrent segmental 'chemical' pneumonia due to aspiration at night.
- *Alcoholics*
    (1) suppression of respiratory reflexes
    (2) diminished defences against infection.
- Occurs with *endobronchial lesions*
    (1) foreign body
    (2) granuloma
    (3) congenital defects
    (4) neoplasm.
- *Post-operative* pneumonias common in smokers especially with a background of chronic chests.
- *Immunological deficits*, either acquired (drugs) or congenital, may result in severe pneumonias (recurrent).
- Incidence rises with *age*.

Pneumococcal pneumonia

> *Pneumococcal pneumonia*
> *features: diagnosis*
>
> - The *most common* bacterial pneumonia
> - Could be *lobar/segmental*
> - Follows a *cold or URTI* (after about 7 days)
> - Herpes simplex (mouth sores) may occur
> - Seen more often in *winter/spring*
> - Onset *abrupt, rigor,* fever, *pleuritic pain* with cough and *'rusty' sputum*. Marked weakness and malaise
>   Tachypnoea/tachycardia: spleen rarely palpable
> - In early stages – signs of constitutional upset only. Later *dullness, bronchial breathing* and *pleural rub*
> - *Sputum* examination *not* necessary unless in doubt
> - *Chest X-ray* (a portable film) (domiciliary) in the very ill will show:
>
>   Right middle, lower lobes commonly involved
>   *Repeat* film after 7–10 days (complete resolution by 6 weeks)
>
> - Leukocyte count *not* indicated unless monitoring response to treatment or using chloramphenicol

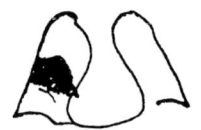

ACUTE INFECTIONS OF THE LUNGS

Pneumococcal pneumonia

Management: Can be at *home* provided:
- a *chest X-ray* can be done
- *frequent supervision* by GP
- patient *not severely ill* (absence of respiratory failure or other disorders)
- home *environment suitable*

General care:
- nurse in warm comfortable position (*propped up at 45°*)
- fluids and electrolyte replacement; give *Re-hidrate*
- *commode* may be needed; leg exercises to prevent DVT

Oxygen:
- in absence of 'chronic chest' – safe to give high concentration (35% via Ventimask up to 8 hours a day)

Analgesics:
- morphine in previously 'fit' individual is safe
- in 'chronic chests', aspirin, paracetamol and dihydrocodeine

Antibiotics:
- 1st choice: benzylpenicillin 1 megaunit twice daily, changing to oral therapy after 2 days and continue for 10 days
- 2nd choice: tetracycline; ampicillin

RESPIRATORY DISEASES

Pneumococcal pneumonia: complications

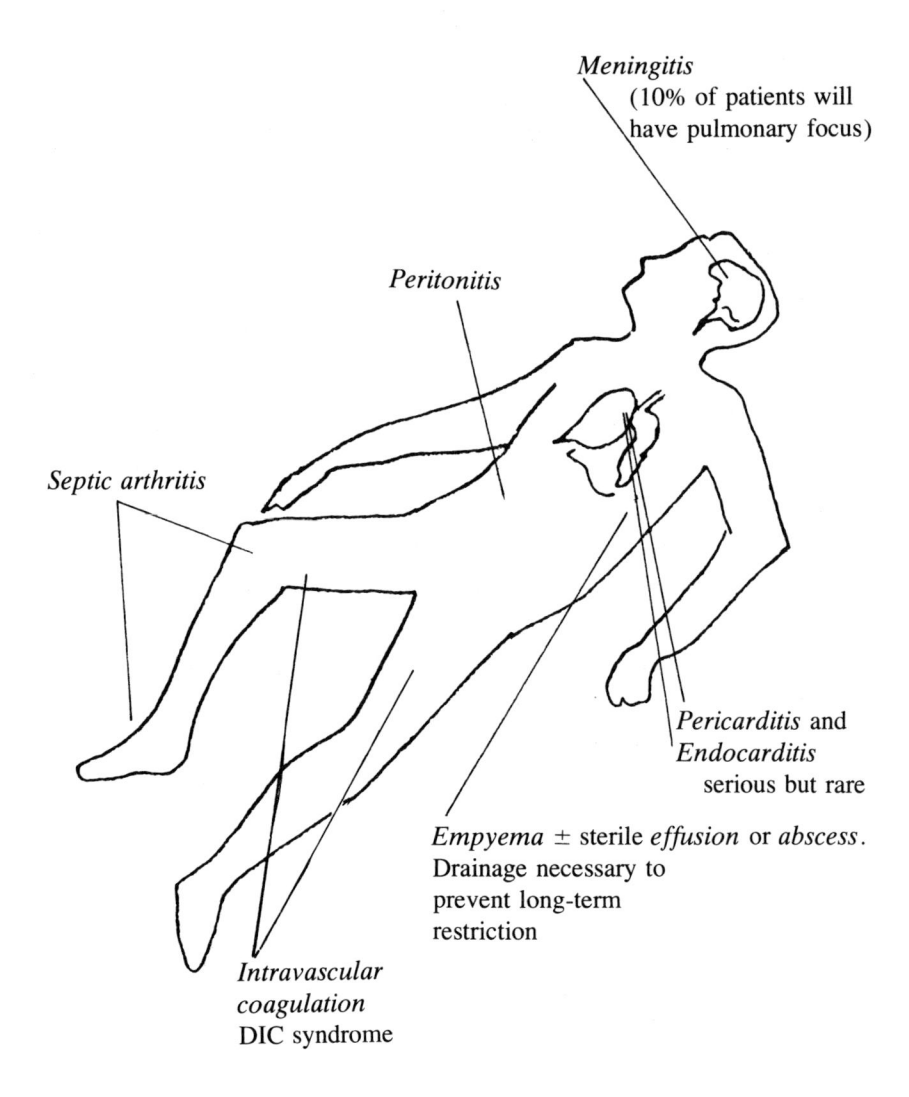

Meningitis (10% of patients will have pulmonary focus)

Peritonitis

Septic arthritis

Pericarditis and *Endocarditis* serious but rare

Empyema ± sterile *effusion* or *abscess*. Drainage necessary to prevent long-term restriction

Intravascular coagulation DIC syndrome

Mortality in elderly and immunological deficient approximately 40–50%

Pneumococcal pneumonia: caution and after-care

Refer to hospital:
- Those with 'chronic chests' with previous history of pneumonia
- At risk of respiratory failure/heart failure
- Insulin dependent diabetics
- Splenectomy: immunosuppressed
- Infarcts/very old
- Failure to respond after 24 hours

After-care:
- See weekly for 4 weeks following initial improvement
- Chest X-ray in 6 weeks – if cleared, return to work
- Those at risk – supply 'antibiotics' to take early in the event of further exacerbation
- Encourage to stop smoking

Bacterial pneumonias (less common)

- Streptococcal

- *Haemophilus influenzae*

- *Staphylococcus*
 (cavitation may occur,
 treat in hospital: *isolation*)
- *Klebsiella* (Friedländer's)

- Suspect in 'influenza' epidemics
 (penicillin)
- In 'chronic' chests
 (ampicillin)
- Alcoholics/aspiration/debilitated
 (flucloxacillin)

- Old, diabetic, alcoholic
- Profuse haemoptysis
- High mortality (50%)
 (cephalosporins)
 (gentamicin)
 (chloramphenicol)

Legionnaire's disease

This is pneumonia due to *Pneumophilus* bacillus

- Identified as explosive outbreak at American Legionnaires' convention in Philadelphia in 1976
- Organisms Gram-negative coccobacillus
- Diagnosis often retrospective

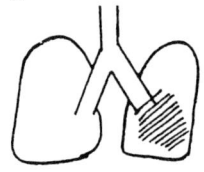

- Resembles viral/mycoplasma pneumonia
- Cough, slight sputum
- Chest X-ray shows lobar consolidation
- High fever, somnolence, diarrhoea, myalgia and bradycardia after about 4–5 days
- DIC may occur
- Special staining for sputum

Use erythromycin 500 mg 6-hourly for 3 weeks
Repeat chest film following treatment. An 'alveolitis' picture may result

Viral pneumonias

- Impossible to diagnose successfully in general practice.
- May coexist with bacterial pneumonias.
- Suspect when rapid dyspnoea and constitutional symptoms. Very little sputum.
- Examination will reveal a very breathless, often cyanosed patient with very few 'chest' signs.
- *Chest X-ray:*

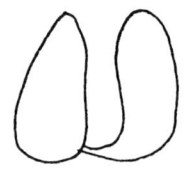

Normal in early stages   Diffuse shadowing – 'white' lung

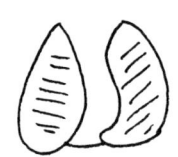

- Treat in hospital. High mortality.

ACUTE INFECTIONS OF THE LUNGS

Chickenpox pneumonia (varicella zoster)

- Chickenpox, a highly contagious childhood problem, may be complicated by pneumonia, encephalitis, myo/pericarditis, hepatitis and renal failure.
- Incidence of varicella pneumonia rises in adults (30%).
- Pulmonary involvement within 5 days after 'rash' – cough, high fever, chest pain, cyanosis and haemoptysis.
- Chest X-ray

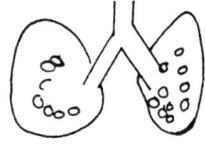

  Widespread nodular opacities; these may calcify later. All adults with varicella should have a chest X-ray.

- Treat in hospital

    oxygen
    ? assisted ventilation
    steroids
    treatment of bacterial complication

Mycoplasma pneumonia

It represents 4% of all pneumonias: 'primary atypical pneumonia'.

- Outbreaks.
- Sore throat; tracheobronchitis; pneumonia.
- Patient is not usually very ill. No signs.
- Chest X-ray may look worse than the patient

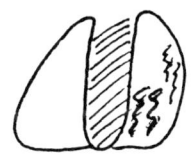

    – patchy infiltrates
    – lower zones
    – unilateral.

- Occasionally complicated by myocarditis, haemolytic anaemia and meningitis.
- Give erythromycin 250–500 mg 6-hourly for 2 weeks or tetracycline.

Cytomegalovirus pneumonia (CMV)

- Endemic prevalence.
- Suspect in immunosuppressed and in association with respiratory distress syndrome (infants).
- Confusion, anoxia, basal crackles.

- *Chest X-ray*

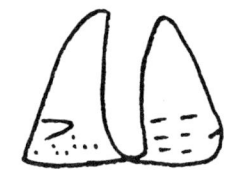

  Basal changes
  Diffuse dense shadows.

- High mortality. No specific therapy.

ACUTE BRONCHITIS

- A *child* may 'suffer' an occasional attack of tracheo-bronchitis – often following a viral infection – and should be treated as acute infective illness.
- *Recurrent acute bronchitis* with *wheeze* may be a pre-runner for bronchial asthma in later years – although many children will not become asthmatic. Difficult to distinguish the two groups, therefore treat *recurrent* acute *wheezy bronchitis* as 'asthma' – *avoid frequent courses* of antibiotics.
- *Adults* with acute bronchitis/bronchiolitis will often have 'chronic chests' and management of acute illness should take into account the underlying disorders and advice offered for these. Wheeze is *not* the main feature of an occasional attack of acute bronchitis.

Acute bronchitis: management

- Treat at home.
- Warm bed, good posture for coughing, fluids.
- Regular aspirin (soluble) – beware in asthma and peptic ulcer – or paracetamol (elixirs in children).
- Oxygen (35%) temporarily : 24–48 hours.
- Breathing exercises. Physiotherapy *not* necessary unless previous history of bronchiectasis.
- When wheezy – give salbutamol tablets or syrup for 5–7 days only.
- Antibiotics (purulent sputum with fever)

  ampicillin
  amoxicillin
  pivampicillin
  (*most cases*)

  Septrin
  cephadrine
  (*penicillin sensitivity*)

ACUTE INFECTIONS OF THE LUNGS

Recurrent acute bronchitis with wheeze: children

- If family or previous history of wheeze or allergy: the child to be regarded asthmatic (*see* Chapter 6, Bronchial Asthma)

- When the diagnosis of asthma not straightforward

  Refer for:
  Specialist assessment

  Give:
  Betasympatho-mimetics, e.g. salbutamol elixir twice a day.

  Theophylline tabs. or elixir at night.

  Oxygen ± nebulizer.

  Steroids: prednisone up to 15 mg/day for 3 days and then reducing over a month. (Only in severe cases)

Antibiotics if definite evidence of infection/bronchiectasis (green sputum and fever)

Yellow sputum may be due to eosinophils etc as in 'asthma'

Recurrent acute bronchitis: adults

- Define the *underlying disorders* – e.g. chronic bronchitis, emphysema, bronchiectasis – and manage as acute exacerbation of COAD (*see* Chapter 5, under Airways Obstruction and Reversibility)

- *Non-smokers* and *those without identifiable 'chronic' disorders* – *refer* for:

  (1) assessment to exclude mechanical problems in the upper/lower respiratory tract, e.g. adenoma, carcinoma; bronchoscopy may be necessary

  (2) ENT assesssment: sinuses, ear-infection and laryngeal lesions

PLEURISY

Types

- Infective (80%) { bacterial / non-bacterial }
- As a result of thromboembolism (5%)
- Post-operative/trauma (2%)
- Due to diseased adjoining organs (spleen, liver, gallbladder)
- Part of systemic condition,
    e.g. Collagen disorders
    Systemic lupus erythematosus
    Systemic sclerosis
    Rheumatoid arthritis
    Polyarteritis nodosa

Pleurisy: management

- Where there is identifiable cause – treat that.
- Patients with suspected pulmonary embolism, trauma (including ruptured spleen) should be referred to hospital.
- Majority of cases of pleurisy secondary to severe lower respiratory tract infection ± pneumonia will respond to treatment of underlying disorders.
- Many will be classed as 'viral pleurodynia' (Börnholm disease):
    (1) reassure
    (2) do *not* use antibiotics
    (3) chest X-ray (if sizeable pleural effusion, refer for advice and assessment)
    (4) keep well hydrated
    (5) adequate analgesics: pethidine, morphine, dihydrocodeine and buprenorphine commonly used
    (6) indomethacin 25 mg 4-hourly for 7–10 days if failure to respond in 48 hours

INFECTED PULMONARY INFARCTION AND SEPTIC EMBOLI

These are *likely to occur specially in:*
- Thromboembolic disease with chronic 'bad' chests
- Immunosuppressed
- Immobility (post-operative, age, on ventilators or in 'plaster')

- Rheumatic valvular heart disease (mitral valve)
- Bacterial endocarditis

Organisms

- Could be especially *Klebsiella*.

Management

Life threatening:
- Treat the underlying condition
- Anticoagulate
- Identify organism and give appropriate antibiotics till the problem resolved

LUNG ABSCESS

What is it?

- It is localized, acute or chronic process of inflammatory origin. There is central necrosis and adjoining pneumonia.
- Commoner in the right lung (the right main bronchus in line with trachea) and most abscesses form following aspiration. These are usually single except in staphylococcal infections.
- Epileptics, alcoholics, post-operative patients more likely.
- Foreign bodies lodging in airways as in dental extraction, tonsillectomy and other ENT procedures may result in sequestration of lung segment and abscess formation.
- Patient with bronchial carcinoma (cavitation).

Organisms isolated

- *Staphylococcus aureus*
- *Klebsiella pneumoniae*
- Anaerobic bacteria
- *Actinomyces*
- *Entamoeba histolytica*

Investigations

Physical signs are few

    episodic fever and rigor, weight loss
    sputum large quantities in some (foul smelling) ± haemoptysis

Chest X-ray

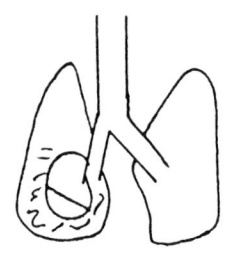

segmental consolidation
+ fluid/air cavity

Complications

These are:

    erosion of a large vessel
    secondary abscess (brain)
    destruction of lung tissue ⟶ bronchiectasis

Lung abscess: management

Get advice from specialist.
    What done?

- *Antibiotics* α-organism and sensitivity
  penicillin oral or parenteral is drug of choice
  metronidazole (rectal or i.v.)
- Postural drainage
- Oxygen and nebulizer therapy when breathless
- When cavity stabilized (on serial chest X-rays) and pneumonitis cleared: bronchoscopy is undertaken (general anaesthetic) in most and using rigid bronchoscope. The procedure should be undertaken where 'surgical' facilities available in case of complication
- Abscess aspirated
- When continued symptoms of cough and sputum in spite of radiological clearing, a repeat bronchoscopy and bronchography necessary

12

Chronic infections of the lungs

☐ ☐ ☐ ☐ ☐ ☐ ☐ ☐ ☐ ☐ ☐ ☐

WHAT ARE THEY?

- Bronchiectasis
- In association with cystic fibrosis of pancreas
- Aspergillosis
- Others

Chronic bronchitis is *not* included here, as strictly it is a diagnosis made on history of cough and sputum (not infected) – usually in winter months only.

BRONCHIECTASIS

This is defined as a condition in which there is a cough and purulent sputum (large quantity) with or without haemoptysis. There may be some reversible airflow obstruction.

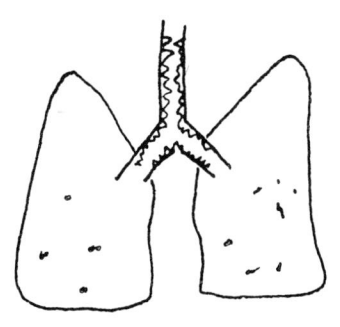

Significance

- Chronic bronchiectasis is usually *permanent* and not to be confused with *transient mild (acute) cylindrical dilatation* of the bronchioles/bronchi which occurs after collapse/consolidation *(pneumonia)*. Recurrent pneumonia of whatever cause may eventually result in destructive, septic disease of the lungs (bronchiectasis).
- The diagnosis is almost always on *history* in early stages.
- *Physical signs* of persistent basal crackles, finger clubbing and failure to thrive are late.
- *Chest X-ray* in mild, early disease is usually *normal*; a *bronchogram* necessary in many for confirmation of diagnosis.
- Coarse crackles (end-inspiratory) heard over the affected part. These may partially 'disappear' or change in intensity as the patient coughs.

Clinical types

Congenital

- Rare
- Extensive (bilateral)
- Early: asymptomatic
- Haemoptysis

(1) Kartagener's sydrome: TRIAD OF:

Absent frontal sinuses
Sinusitis

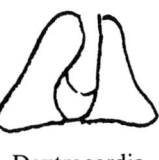

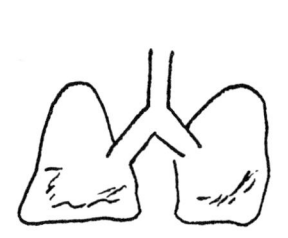

Dextrocardia   Bronchiectasis

(2) With *cystic fibrosis (see below)* (mucoviscidosis)
(3) With congenital *kyphoscoliosis*
(4) *Tracheobronchomegaly*: dilatation of main (large) airways.

Acquired disease

- More common
- Often localized
- Significant symptoms
- Airways obstruction in many
- History of TB, asthma and chronic bronchitis (especially in children)
- Haemoptysis – less than in congenital

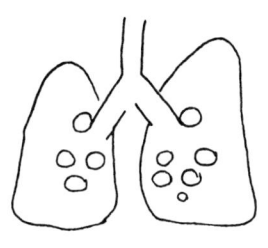

Types
(1)

- Marked dilatation of main airways or perihilar cysts
- Obstruction less likely

(2)

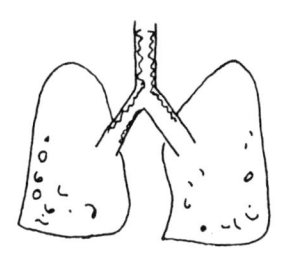

- Less dilated airways
- Interstitial lung disease
- Airways obstruction likely

RESPIRATORY DISEASES

Features

• Failure to thrive (children)	• Anorexia, weight loss and general debility common
• Anaemia	• Usually normocytic – normochromic
• Finger clubbing	• ± Cyanosis
• Dyspnoea	• Constant with exacerbation. Wheeze may suggest reversible airways obstruction
• Neurological syndromes – headaches, confusion and fits	• As a result of secondary cerebral abscess
• Kidney involvement 'Amyloidosis'	• In rare cases nephrotic syndrome occurs – proteinuria enough to cause hypoproteinaemia and oedema

Problems

- How to confirm the diagnosis?
- Is sputum examination indicated?
- Whom to refer for surgery?
- Prophylactic therapy – what?
- Physiotherapy/patient education?

Bronchogram ± bronchoscopy

- A chest X-ray in *established cases* of *mild* to *moderate* disease will show peribronchial shadowing with cavities in the 'dependent' areas. Repeat yearly to see the progression.

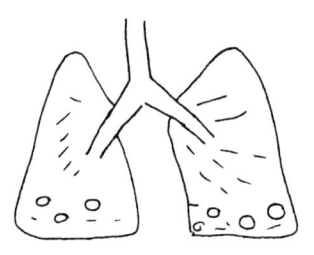

Reticulocavitating shadowing – mainly at the lung bases.
Hyperinflation seen where there is a degree of airways obstruction

- In a patient with chronic symptoms where the chest X-ray is normal – bronchoscopy indicated. The operator will invariably undertake bronchography.
- *Bronchogram* will show:
  (1) Extent of disease: unilateral/bilateral
  (2) Type: cylindrical/cystic
  (3) Dilatation of main airways

Sputum examination

- Assessment of *volume* (24 hours), *type* of material expectorated is more important. Large amount (over 1 cupful a day) and haemoptysis need further assessment in hospital ⟶ refer to a chest physician.
- *'Foul' smelling* sputum indicates acute exacerbation and specimen to be sent for culture. *Lung abscess* may be present.
- *'Glue-like', thick green* material may suggest complication with *aspergillus*. In these cases ask for a special laboratory staining for 'mycelium'.
- Check regularly for *AAFB* if *previous history of TB*.
- If a patient is a *smoker*, send for *malignant cells*.

Surgery

Aim at a 'cure'.

- Patient should first be referred to a physician for

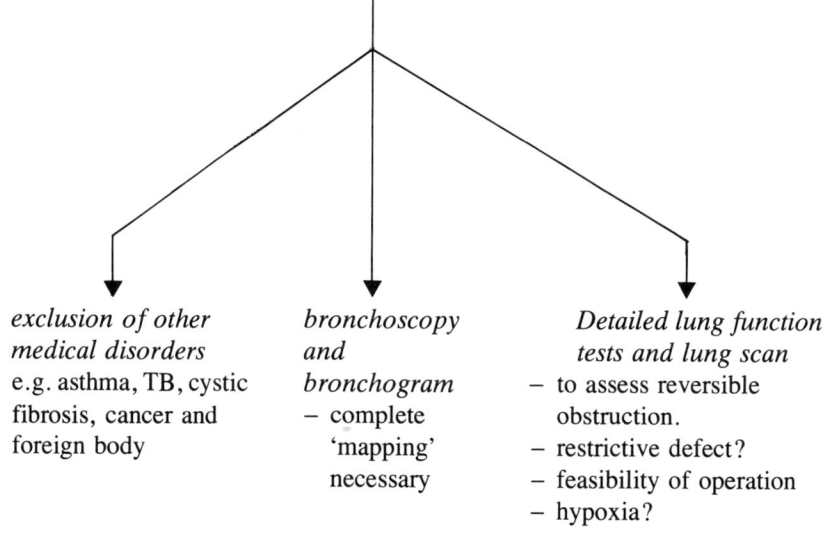

| *exclusion of other medical disorders* e.g. asthma, TB, cystic fibrosis, cancer and foreign body | *bronchoscopy and bronchogram* – complete 'mapping' necessary | *Detailed lung function tests and lung scan* – to assess reversible obstruction. – restrictive defect? – feasibility of operation – hypoxia? |

RESPIRATORY DISEASES

- Surgical treatment usually in *localized* disease only – in a young otherwise healthy individual.

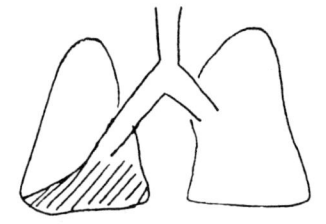

Operative mortality in selected cases very low (1.5%)

Limited pathology ⟶ removal of a segment or a lobe.
Results: up to 50% completely cured after limited resection (10-year follow-up)[1].

Drug therapy

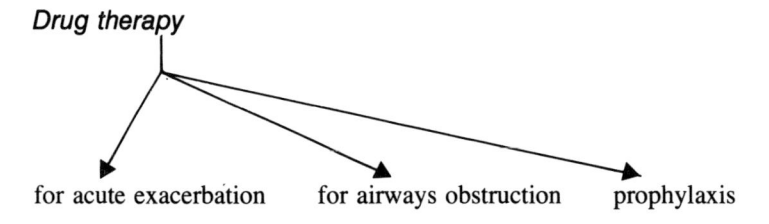

for acute exacerbation   for airways obstruction   prophylaxis

Acute exacerbation

This may follow upper respiratory tract 'viral' illness, influenza or sinusitis. Special risk after anaesthetic including dental treatment. Laboratory examination of sputum *not* helpful.

- Likely organisms:
  Haemophilus influenzae
  Pneumococcus
  Pseudomonas (rare)
  ('foul' smelling sputum)

- Give:
  ampicillin
  or
  amoxicillin
  } 250 mg 6-hourly for 7 days

- Oxygen and nebulizer in 'chronic cases'
- Keep warm/hydrate
- Arrange domiciliary physiotherapy and drainage
- Expectorants *not* indicated
- Salbutamol oral or syrup when significant wheeze

Associated airways obstruction

- Exclude bronchial asthma
  - Family history of allergy
  - Previous asthma
  - High eosinophil count
  - Asthma stigmata in sputum
- Assess degree of reversibility
  - PEFR before and after treatment
  - Note objective improvement in signs with increased exercise tolerance
  - Improved blood P_{O_2}, P_{CO_2}
- Trial of drugs (absence of asthma)
  - Sympathomimetic *inhalers* salbutamol, fenoterol, terbutaline 3 or 4 times a day
  - *Oral* theophyllines and SR aminophylline
    (Phyllocontin)
    (Slophyllin)
  - *Oral* sympathomimetic, salbutamol (Spandet) 8 mg nocte
  - Nebulized therapy 2 or 3 times a day
  - Oral prednisone 5 mg b.d. for 4 weeks

  Do *not* give inhaled steroid.

Prophylactic therapy: in moderate to severe cases

- When symptoms worse during winter months
  (1) *Kelfizine-W* 2 g per week between September and April
      (a) Well tolerated by most
      (b) Encourage fluids
      (c) Effective
      (d) May precipitate gout
  (2) *Septrin* 1 or 2 tabs daily for 2 days in a week. (Gastrointestinal upset common.)
  (3) Tetracycline 250 mg 6-hourly for 2 days in a week.

Sputum sensitivity necessary only if failure to respond.

- If symptoms all year

   Courses of ampicillin, cephalosporins, Septrin, tetracycline, erythromycin or Kelfizine-W.

   According to sputum sensitivity – to be undertaken every 4 weeks.

Physiotherapy (postural drainage)

- Very useful as there is loss of lung elasticity and *bronchiectasis affects the dependent zones.*
- Initially seek advice from a physiotherapist – tell her to *'concentrate' on affected lobes.*
- *Request* that the *patient/relatives* be *educated* especially in postural drainage.
- Ask whether *nebulized therapy* would *ease* the task of *expectoration* in some.

CHRONIC LUNG SEPSIS WITH CYSTIC FIBROSIS OF PANCREAS

What is it?

- Autosomal recessive. When both parents are carriers, there is 1:4 chance of cystic fibrotic child.

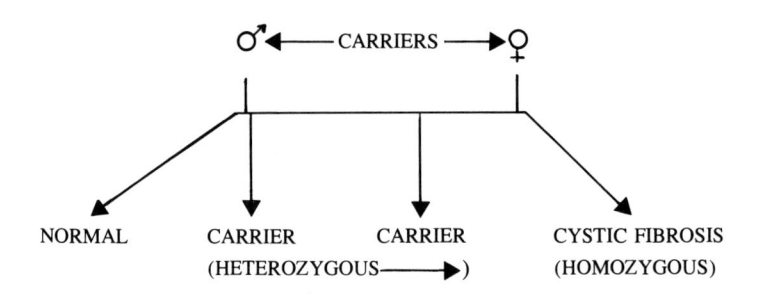

```
            ♂ ◄──── CARRIERS ────► ♀
            │                      │
    ┌───────┼──────────┬───────────┤
    ▼       ▼          ▼           ▼
 NORMAL  CARRIER    CARRIER   CYSTIC FIBROSIS
         (HETEROZYGOUS ────►)   (HOMOZYGOUS)
```

- Relatively common (2–5:10 000 births) childhood disorder continuing in adult life.
- Although may involve many systems, the pancreas and the lungs most important.
- Sweat is hypertonic (increased Na^+ and Cl^-) – basis for the 'sweat' test.
- There is marked hypertrophy of mucosal glands in the chest.

CHRONIC INFECTIONS OF THE LUNGS

Pathology

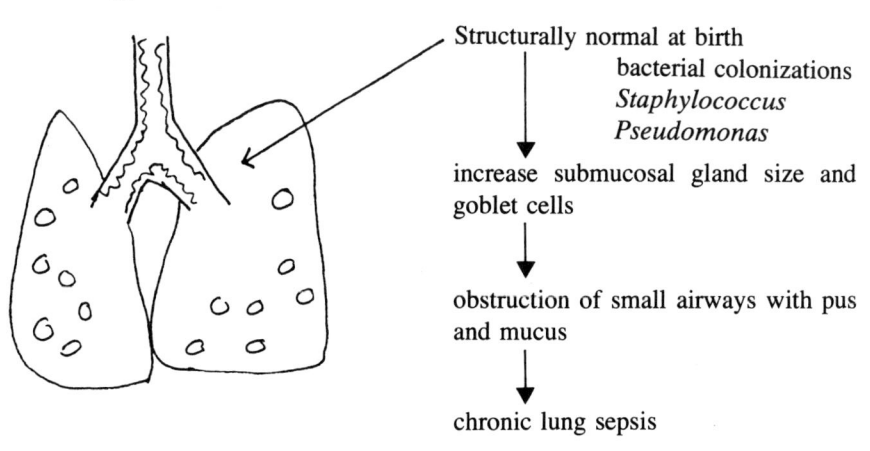

Structurally normal at birth
    ↓ bacterial colonizations
    Staphylococcus
    Pseudomonas

increase submucosal gland size and goblet cells

↓

obstruction of small airways with pus and mucus

↓

chronic lung sepsis

Features

- Normal at birth: therefore escape detection
- Elevated sweat electrolytes: 'salty taste' on kissing
- Hyperinflated chest
- Failure to thrive
- Bulky, offensive stools

- Except when meconium ileus is present
- From birth
- Hypoproteinaemia, anaemia and jaundice
- Bruising/vitamin K deficiency

Management

General principles:

- *Asymptomatic* children may *not* need any *specific treatment*.
- All children should be referred to a *paediatrician* initially.
- *Special units* for treatment and assessment where the child/parents/GPs will obtain advice on future care including schooling.
- Those who *survive the childhood* years will eventually be referred to a *physician*.
- Aim to treat the patient at home with *infrequent visits to outpatients*. However some children will need repeated hospital admissions.
  *Special risk of acquiring antibiotic resistant infections.

Specific treatment

Aims

- Reduce the tenacity and quantity of sputum.
- Prevent secondary infection.
- Identify cases suitable for nebulizer therapy.
- Identify those for prophylactic antibiotic therapy – oral or inhaled?
- Replace pancreatic enzymes.
- Normal education and lifestyle if possible.
- Adequate nutrition.
- Prevent smoking.

Postural drainage

- This is *distressing* and *inconvenient* for the child.
- A *good rapport* with a physiotherapist is important.
- *Same person* should treat if possible, and parents be educated at an early stage.
- Very young infants treated on the lap, but older children prefer tilted beds.

Antibiotics

- Most antibiotics are safe.
- Favoured choices include:
  cephalosporins
  erythromycin
  ampicillin/amoxicillin
- Severe exacerbation may need gentamicin ± treatment of anaerobes.
- Laboratory examination of sputum every 3 months useful – if possible vary the choice of antibiotics according to culture results of organism identified.

Complications

- Extensive destructive lung disease with fibrosis and aspergillosis
- Lung abscess
- Pneumothorax
- Sterility (♂)

CHRONIC INFECTIONS OF THE LUNGS

Prognosis

- Improvement in treatment and early identification of cases will improve the outlook.
- Each individual will vary in the future outlook, therefore do not be specific about prognosis.
- *Death* usually from respiratory failure.

ASPERGILLOSIS

Significance

- *Ubiquitous* in nature. Grain heavily contaminated with aspergillus spores – farm workers at a special risk. *Aspergillus fumigatus* and *A. niger* commonly responsible in human disease.
- Extrapulmonary infections include
  (1) ears (otomycosis),
  (2) finger nails (onychomycosis),
  (3) meningitis.
- *Aspergillus* can be a *contaminant* in the sputum. *No reliable test* to show significant disease. Positive sputum and skin test and precipitins in the serum necessary.
- It may *complicate* TB, cancer, asthma and lung fibrosis (alveolitis). Rarely in postinfluenzal (viral) pneumonia, and in *immunosuppressed* patient, an *invasive*, fatal form described[2].

Clinical types

- *Asthmatic syndrome*

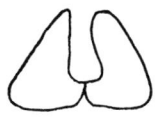

  Hyperinflation

- *Indistinguishable* from *allergic asthma* due to other antigens

- *Acute pneumonitis*

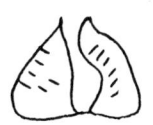

  Upper lobe infiltration

- *Farmers' lung* (*see* Chapter 13, under Occupational Diseases)

- *Bronchopulmonary disease*

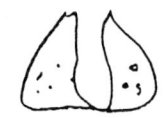

  Transient infiltrates mainly upper lobes.

  – Skin tests and precipitin positive in up to 80%

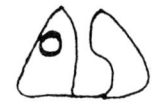

- *Mycetoma*

  Fungal ball complicating a cavity

  Classical X-ray (ask for tomogram)

- *Asthma and pulmonary eosinophilia* common in UK (October–February)

- *Previous history* of TB, cancer, histoplasmosis and bronchiectasis. *Haemorrhage* may occur (erosion of a vessel)

Management

- Those with *asthma syndromes* including

  pneumonitis
  bronchopulmonary disease
  invasive disease

- Give *bronchodilators*
- *Inhalation* (daily) of brilliant green (2-hydroxystilbamidine) and natamycin useful in severe chronic disease
- *Clotrimazole* still under trial stages. Worth using in severe cases
- *Corticosteroids* (oral prednisone) necessary to prevent damage. Maintenance dose 5–7.5 mg daily for 2–3 years. Monitor dose α-eosinophil count (keep under 400)
- *Amphotericin B* (infusion) $\pm$ *5-fluorocytosine* in invasive disease. Side-effects:
  (1) renal failure
  (2) hypokalaemia
  (3) high fever

- *Mycetoma (aspergilloma)*

- Try clotrimazole and amphotericin
- If good lung function – refer for surgical removal

CHRONIC INFECTIONS OF THE LUNGS

OTHER MYCOSES

- *Moniliasis* (rare):
  In malignant disease, diabetes, steroids, malnutrition.

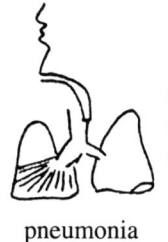

  oral, pharyngeal plaques with *Candida albicans*

  pneumonia

- Ill patient with fever and signs of pneumonia
- In *significant disease* give nystatin or amphotericin lozenges to clear mouth:
  nystatin inhalation
  amphotericin B (i.v.)

- *Actinomycoses:*
  Non-contagious, chronic, granulomatous lung disease

  mimic TB
  soft tissue abscess with empyema/pneumonia

  'ray fungus' – H & E staining and 'sulphur granules'

- Jaw ('lumpy jaw') with abscesses and sinuses of the skin and chest wall
- *Penicillin* for 2–3 months; if allergic give erythromycin
- Good prognosis

- *Cryptococcus:*

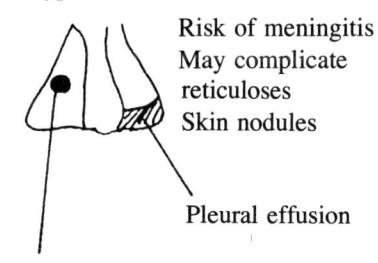

  Risk of meningitis
  May complicate reticuloses
  Skin nodules

  Pleural effusion

  Dense lesion

- Amphotericin B (i.v.)
- Clotrimazole
- ? Rifampicin

- *Histoplasmosis*
  localised or disseminated[3]

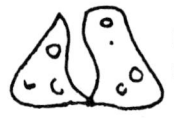

  Pneumonic lesions
  miliary disease

- May have 'granulomatous' lesions especially in the tongue, liver, spleen
- Invasive/pneumonic disease: give amphotericin-B (i.v.) and hydrocortisone to relieve hypersensitivity effects of amphotericin

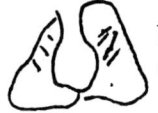

  Upper lobe disease

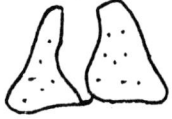

  Widespread calcification

  Common in parts of America

- *Coccidioidomycosis and blastomycosis* (rare in UK):

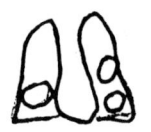

- Ampotericin B

References
1. Clark, N. S. (1965). *Br. Med. J.*, **1,** 80
2. Jariwalla, A. G. et al. (1980). *Thorax*, **35,** 215
3. Jariwalla, A. G. et al. (1977). *Br. Med. J.*, **1,** 1000

13

Fibrotic lung disorders

☐ ☐ ☐ ☐ ☐ ☐ ☐ ☐ ☐ ☐ ☐ ☐

WHAT ARE THEY?

(1) Occupational diseases
(2) Drug-induced conditions
(3) Disorders associated with collagen disease
(4) Cryptogenic
(5) Sarcoidosis (*see* Chapter 10)

OCCUPATIONAL DISEASES

Pneumoconiosis

Diseases characterized by lung damage due to inhalation of organic/inorganic dusts.

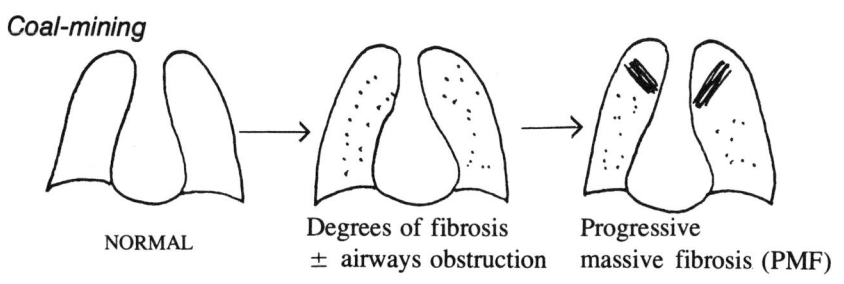

Coal-mining

NORMAL → Degrees of fibrosis ± airways obstruction → Progressive massive fibrosis (PMF)

500 new cases diagnosed (1978) in UK (as reported to pneumoconiosis panel)
N.B. *Caplan's syndrome:* rheumatoid nodules in the lungs of a miner with pneumoconiosis.

Asbestos-induced

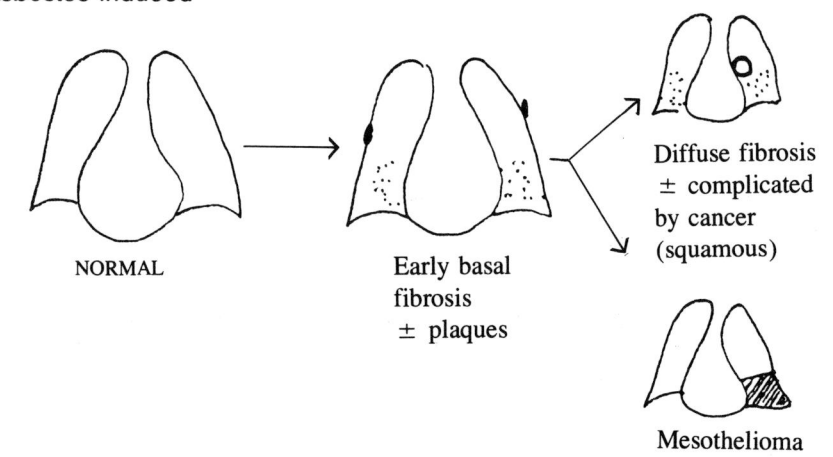

NORMAL → Early basal fibrosis ± plaques

Diffuse fibrosis ± complicated by cancer (squamous)

Mesothelioma

200 new cases of asbestosis (without mesothelioma) (1978) in UK.
200 new cases of mesothelioma (1978) in UK (1:4 with asbestosis).

Other dusts

Silica

Acute illness following heavy exposure over a short duration.

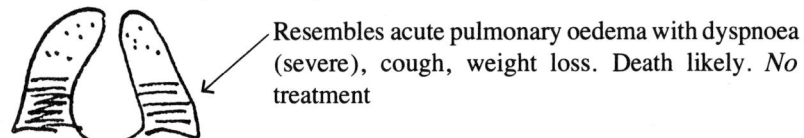

Resembles acute pulmonary oedema with dyspnoea (severe), cough, weight loss. Death likely. *No treatment*

Chronic illness:

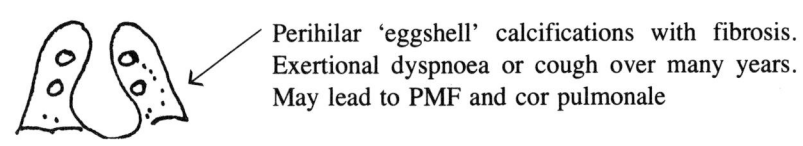

Perihilar 'eggshell' calcifications with fibrosis. Exertional dyspnoea or cough over many years. May lead to PMF and cor pulmonale

Beryllium

- One or two new cases diagnosed in UK per year
- Used in alloy, ceramic industries
- Housewives may be affected dealing with husbands' clothes

FIBROTIC LUNG DISORDERS

Acute illness: heavy exposure

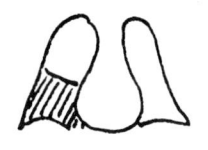

Pneumonia
Breathlessness, haemoptysis
→ Oxygen, steroids useful
Some will progress to respiratory failure

Chronic illness:

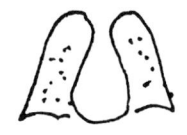

- Granulomatous, systemic disease
- Progressive dyspnoea and dry cough
- Rare
- Patch test *not* diagnostic

Nodular, fibrotic lesions may precede symptoms. Indistinguishable from alveolitis, especially *sarcoid*

plus
Hepatosplenomegaly

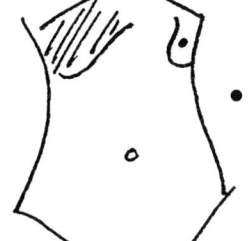

- give steroids
  - *alleviates* symptoms
  - *prolongs life* (maintenance therapy necessary in majority)
  - *complete remission* is described

Management of all forms of pneumoconiosis

- Detailed occupational history
- Include spouse's work and wartime pursuits
- Chest X-rays – if normal, repeat annually
- If abnormal, refer to Chest Clinic – pneumoconiosis panel
- Lung function tests (detailed)
- Will show restrictive defect and diminutions of transfer factor
- Any complications, e.g. cor pulmonale
- Treat with oxygen and diuretics

Mesothelioma

- First associated with asbestos in mid-1940s – conclusively proven in 1960 (Wagner, J. C. et al. (1960). *Br. J. Indust. Med.*, **17,** 260)
- Usually a long period between exposure and disease (average 15–20 years)
- Crocidolite (blue) type most implicated
- No definite association with cigarette smoking

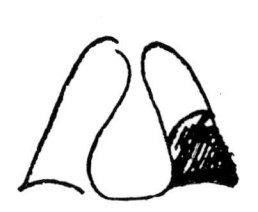

Features

- Pleural > peritoneal
- Either sex but ♂ > ♀
- Occupational or incidental
- Risk increases with degree and duration of exposure
- Common in *blue* and *brown* form

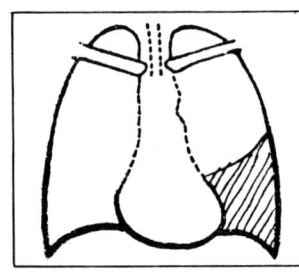

Findings

- *Insidious* onset of symptoms
- *Constant* chest pain, dyspnoea
- Pleural effusion
- Diagnosis: pleural/open biopsy. Often difficult

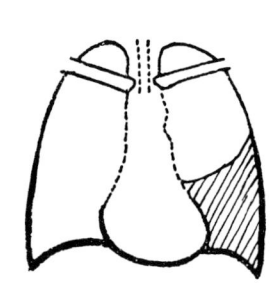

Management

- Symptomatic. Refer to a specialist
- Relieve pain (morphine – oral or parenteral)
- Give adequate oxygen
- Sedatives + analgesics as difficulty in sleeping due to pain
- *No* benefit from radiotherapy, surgery or chemotherapy
- Average survival 12–15 months

Further reading:

Hillerdal, G. (1983). Malignant mesothelioma 1982. Review of 4710 published cases. *Br. J. Dis. Chest*, **77,** 321

Law, M. R. *et al.* (1984). *Thorax,* **39,** 255-9

Farmers' lung (allergic alveolitis)

- Due to inhalation of organic dusts (mouldy hay)
- Commonly the antigen – *Micropolyspora faeni*

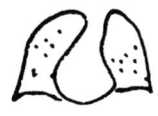

	Features
Acute: faint opacities	• Wheezing (rare), fever, cough and dyspnoea common • Cyanosis • Widespread crackles • Reappearance of symptoms and signs on re-exposure
Chronic diffuse honey-combing	• Severe exertional dyspnoea • *No* eosinophilia in blood or sputum • *No* reliable test • Respiratory and cardiac failure (cor pulmonale) lead to early death

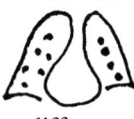

Management
• Prevention – dry the hay, adequate ventilation   • 'Risk' group to avoid recurring exposure   • Seek alternative employment, especially in one-man farm   • *Give* large doses of steroids (prednisone) in acute cases

DRUGS AND THE LUNGS

- Estimated 5% of patients given 'drugs' will manifest allergic or hypersensitivity reactions
- Adopt a high index of suspicion
- Only the 'common' types described here (a detailed account is given by Durant, J. R. et al. (1979). *Cleve. Clin. Q.*, **46**

Hypersensitivity (asthmatic syndromes)

- Cough, wheeze, dyspnoea
- Eosinophilia

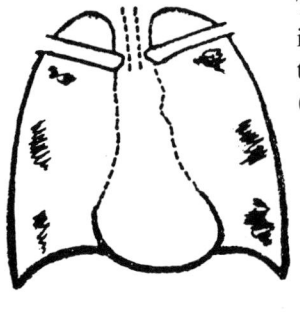

Transient infiltrates of the lungs (periphery)

- Stop the drug
- Give 2–3 weeks course of steroids – prednisone (initially 45 mg/day) in severe reactions
- Inform Committee on Safety of Medicines

- *Types:* azathioprine
  busulphan
  bleomycin
  carbamazepine
  penicillamine
  PAS
  isoniazid

Pneumonitis/fibrosis

- Features similar to hypersensitivity reactions
- Disease *more* chronic

SLE syndrome

- Remove the drug (resolution may take up to 3 months)
- Use corticosteroids if severe constitutional symptoms as well

- *Types:* bleomycin
  amiodarone
  methyldopa
  hydrallazine
  'the pill'
  procainamide
  nitrogen mustard
  procarbazine

FIBROTIC LUNG DISORDERS

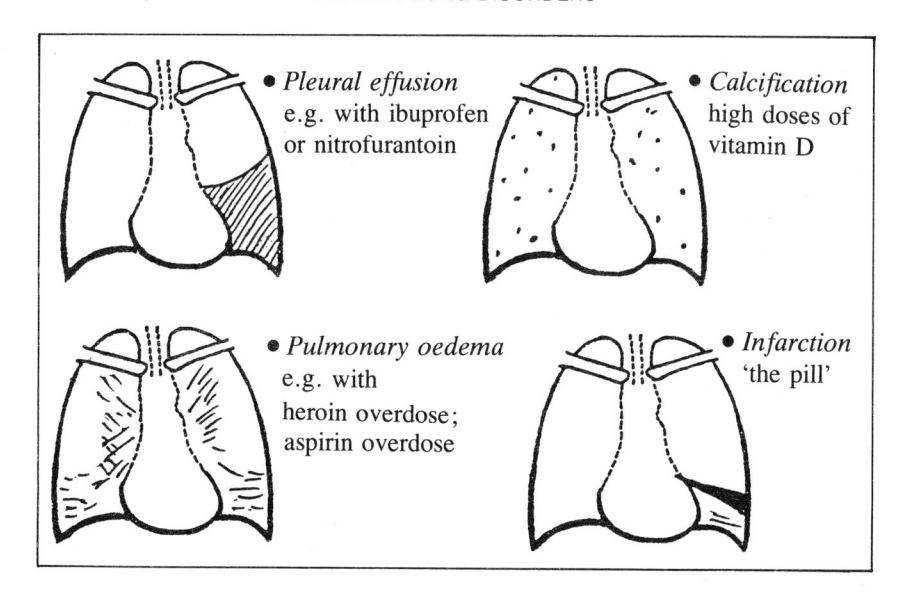

- *Pleural effusion*
  e.g. with ibuprofen
  or nitrofurantoin

- *Calcification*
  high doses of
  vitamin D

- *Pulmonary oedema*
  e.g. with
  heroin overdose;
  aspirin overdose

- *Infarction*
  'the pill'

COLLAGEN DISORDERS AND THE LUNGS

Rheumatoid arthritis

Treat underlying conditions; steroids useful.

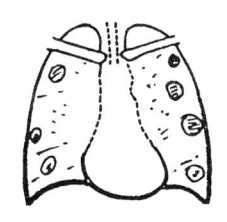

Peripheral nodules

Caplan's syndrome:

- Spherical (1–5 cm), peripheral lesions, i.e. nodules in a patient with rheumatoid arthritis who is a miner. Lesions may cavitate.
  Increased risk for tuberculosis

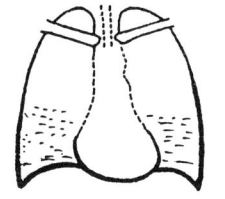

Basal increased reticulations

Alveolitis:

- May be indistinguishable from cryptogenic alveolitis. Look for evidence of seropositive arthritis ± Sjögren's syndrome (keratoconjunctivitis)

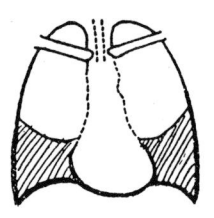

RESPIRATORY DISEASES

Effusion

- May be large and bilateral
- Low level of sugar in the fluid aspirated
- May need recurrent aspirations and pleurodesis if no response to drug (steroid) therapy

Pleural effusion

Systemic lupus erythematosus

Refer for assessment and advice on future care.

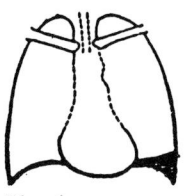

Pleurisy/thickening:

- May be transient. Severe pain may mimic pulmonary embolism, especially when on steroids

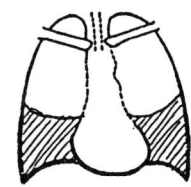

Pleurisy

Unilateral/bilateral pleural effusion:

- May be complicated by pneumothorax/hydropneumothorax
- Pleurectomy may be necessary

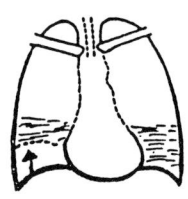

Effusions

Basal collapse/fibrosis:

- Patient breathless
- Diaphragm may be raised
- Severe disability – needing long term steroids and oxygen

Scleroderma

Detailed general assessment necessary.

- Usually a female between 30 and 50 years of age
- Other systemic features evident
- Over 30% with lung involvement

FIBROTIC LUNG DISORDERS

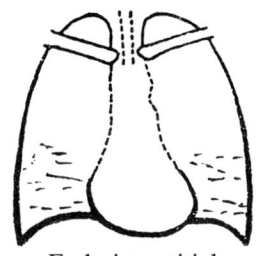

Early interstitial fibrosis

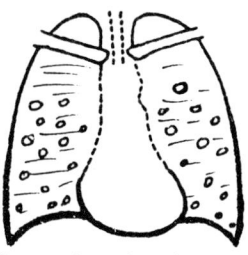

Severe lung involvement with honeycombing

- Breathlessness
- Cough
- Recurrent infections ± pneumonia
- Respiratory failure
- May be complicated by adenocarcinoma

Polyarteritis nodosa

Rare. Refer for initial assessment.

- Lung involvement in about 30%
- *Suspect when:*

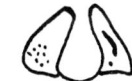

    (1) – flitting lung shadows
    – small bilateral pleural effusions

    (2) High ESR: 70 – often above 100

    (3) Very high eosinophil count (often over 2500–5000)

    (4) High blood pressure

- May cause recurrent asthma
- Muscle biopsy/lung biopsy to confirm diagnosis
- Demonstration of 'aneurysms'
- *Give* prednisone initially 45 mg/day, reducing over a period of 4 weeks with response monitored on signs, symptoms and lowering of ESR and eosinophils

    Maintenance dose 5–7.5 mg daily

- *Prognosis:* Better survival rates on steroids as opposed to without (Frohnert, P. P. (1967) *Am. J. Med.*, **43,** 8)

Wegener's granulomatosis

A rare condition.
- Granulomatous disorder

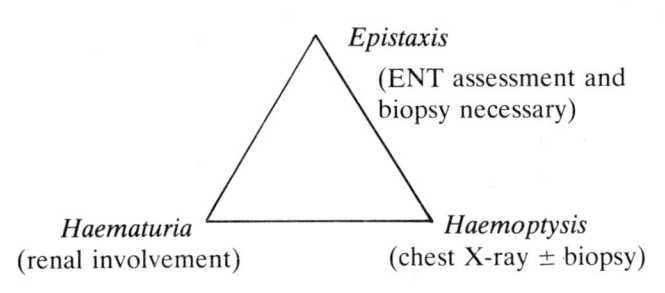

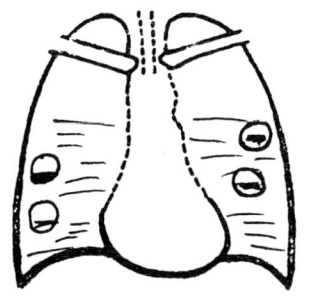

Epistaxis
(ENT assessment and biopsy necessary)

Haematuria
(renal involvement)

Haemoptysis
(chest X-ray ± biopsy)

-

Chest X-ray: mid-zone, cavitating, rounded lesion with fibrosis

- Treatment: difficult. Refer for assessment to a specialized unit

  STEROIDS ± Immunosuppression ± Cytotoxics

- *Prognosis* with lung and kidney involvement: Very Poor

FIBROSING ALVEOLITIS (HAMMAN–RICH SYNDROME)

- *Aetiology unknown.*
- *Histological* diagnosis *essential* as there is variable response to treatment of different types, therefore refer for assessment to a chest physician.

FIBROTIC LUNG DISORDERS

- *Features*

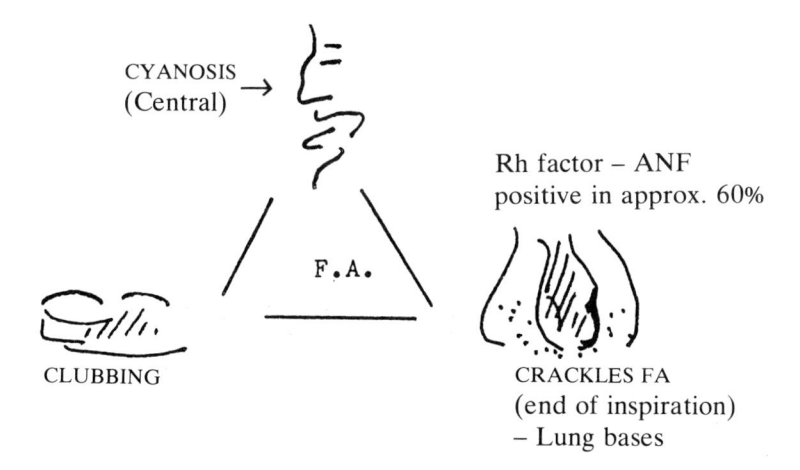

CYANOSIS (Central)

CLUBBING

F.A.

Rh factor – ANF positive in approx. 60%

CRACKLES FA
(end of inspiration)
– Lung bases

- *Restrictive defect on lung function tests*

  FEV_1 (reduced)   *Low* transfer factor
  but ratio 80/90
  FVC (reduced)   *Low* coefficient

- *Prognosis:* Poor. Die in respiratory failure.

Management of fibrosing alveolitis

- Use *steroids* in most; prednisone 45 mg a day for 2 weeks; then gradually reducing to maintenance 5–7.5 mg daily
  Response better in:
  no fibrosis histologically

- *Cyclophosphamide* and *azathioprine*
  (better in conjunction with a small dose of prednisone)

- ? *Penicillamine*

- Assess objective improvement: increased exercise tolerance improved lung function tests improved blood gases

- Use when high dose steroid regime not effective

- Effectiveness not established

14

Emergencies

☐☐☐☐☐☐☐☐☐☐☐☐

WHAT ARE THEY?

- Severe acute asthma
- Pneumothorax
- Acute exacerbation of chest including pneumonia
- Severe croup
- Epiglottitis
- Injuries
- Acute 'white' lung syndromes
- Pulmonary embolus/infarction (Chapter 2)

SPONTANEOUS PNEUMOTHORAX

• Type of patient	• Tall, slim smoker:
• Seasonal variation	• None
• Existing lung disease	• Asthma, TB, cancer and fibrosis
• Features (In small lesion there are no symptoms)	• Sudden increase in dyspnoea with pleuritic chest pain. Suspect when patient, e.g. with asthma, fails to respond to therapy. Clinical signs are unhelpful

- Ask for chest X-ray in expiration/ inspiration to show the extent of 'collapse'

  Showing approx. 20% collapse of one lung

- Repeat film *soon after intubation* OR if treated *conservatively* after 3 days

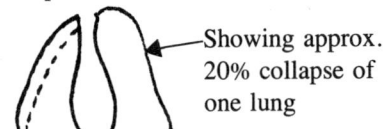

- Recurrence

- Pneumothorax may recur 1:4

Management

At home

- Young, healthy non-smoker
- Less than one third collapse of one lung
- Relatively little discomfort with pain and dyspnoea
- Facilities of immediate chest X-ray and admission if necessary
- Daily supervision possible
- Advice from specialist ± physiotherapy

What to do:
- Explain the problem to patient and relative
- Analgesics regularly
- Antibiotics if infection
- 'Breathing' exercises 3×20 min a day
- If chest X-ray shows complete re-expansion ⟶ work

In hospital

- Pre-existing disease of the lungs especially asthma and emphysema. (A very small degree of collapse would be devastating)
- Collapse > one third of a lung
- Previous history of pneumothorax
- Lack of supervision and facilities for urgent admission
- Those who 'fail' home treatment (after 24–36 hours)

What done?

- 2nd intercostal space
- Argyll-cannula or 'rubber' tube
- Underwater seal

In recurrence or continual leak, attempt *'medical' pleurodesis* using talc or tetracycline (1.5 g)

↓

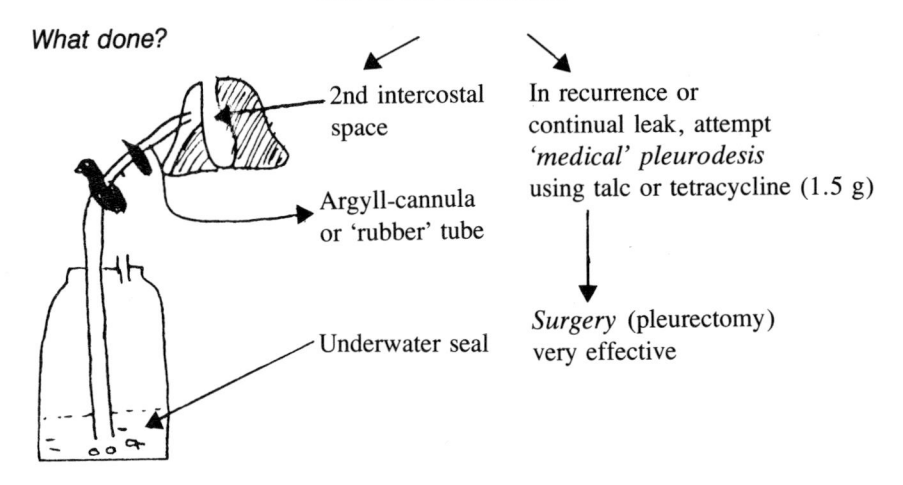

Surgery (pleurectomy) very effective

TENSION PNEUMOTHORAX

- Type of patient
- Previous history

- Features

- Chest X-ray (very essential)
  - Trachea
  - Hyperlucent area. Usually no significant shift of trachea in congenital cysts

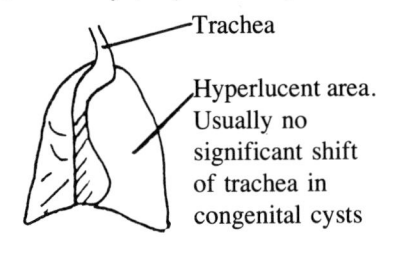

- Any
- Stabbing, road traffic accident, resuscitation (cardiac), pleural aspiration
- Respiratory distress (severe); cyanosis; deviated trachea. Electrocardiogram (if available): right axis deviation
- Try inserting a needle with a moist syringe on the hyper-resonant side: the plunger will be pushed out

- *Treatment in hospital*
  (1) Intercostal drainage with 'pressure'
  (2) May need assisted ventilation

INJURIES TO CHEST

- Commonly in road traffic accidents
- Other organs commonly involved
- Look for bruises over the chest wall
- Patient may become acutely breathless and complain of severe chest pain
- Paradoxical movement of the chest
- Result in disturbance of ventilation – head injury and debris in bronchial passages will aggravate the situation.

Types

> Rib fractures
> Flail chest
> Lung contusion and laceration
> Pleural damage

Immediate management

- Careful examination and notes on injury (*chest X-ray necessary*)

> *Front:*
> Depressions of the chest wall (stove-in chest)
> Paradoxical movement
> Shift of mediastinum
>
> *Back:*
> BRUISES
> SWELLING

- Treatment

> Clear the passages
> Relieve pain with morphine
> Tracheostomy may be necessary
> Stabilize chest wall (strapping)
> 'Escort' to hospital

ACUTE RESPIRATORY FAILURE

- Defined as a state when lung ventilation and perfusion inadequate and resulting in hypercapnia (high P_{CO_2}) and hypoxia (low P_{O_2}), therefore can only be firmly diagnosed on blood gas estimation.
- *Causes:*

> Acute on chronic chest diseases including bronchitis and asthma
> Viral/bacterial pneumonia
> Inhalation of irritants and foreign body
> Massive pulmonary embolus
> Neurological, e.g. Guillain–Barré syndrome
> Injuries
> Septicaemia

Diagnosis

- *Increase in breathlessness:*
  A 'disabled' person will become more breathless in an effort to maintain near normal blood gases.
- *Decrease in respiratory effort:*
  An asthmatic patient – especially the elderly – will be exhausted leading to poor effort in breathing. This will result in high P_{CO_2}. These patients often need assisted ventilation.
- *Drowsiness, confusion, twitching, convulsions, pain:*
  (1) These are features of respiratory failure.
  (2) Occasionally worsened by 'sedatives' given to chronic chest patients.
  (3) Pain may suggest pulmonary embolus or pneumothorax.
- *Cyanosis, flapping tremor of hands and raised intracranial pressure:*
  Initial bounding pulse and warm peripheries due to hypercapnia will result in poor volume fast pulse (hypoxia).

Dangers

- Respiratory failure especially in chronic chest patients carries a high mortality, therefore treat in hospital.
- Chest X-ray, electrocardiograph and blood gases necessary.

Assisted ventilation often necessary in

> - Elderly *asthmatics*
> - Those with deteriorating *neurological illness*
> - Severe *pulmonary oedema*
> - *Multiple injuries*

- 'Others'

> A small pneumothorax may cause devastation in chronic chest ⟶ intercostal drainage
>
> Bronchoscopy (rigid) for inhalation, e.g. foreign body
>
> Anticoagulants/surgery for pulmonary thrombosis

Multiple Choice Questions

☐ ☐ ☐ ☐ ☐ ☐ ☐ ☐ ☐ ☐ ☐

(1) A previously healthy young individual develops acute dyspnoea and chest pain. The following most likely:
- (a) pneumothorax
- (b) sarcoidosis
- (c) cor pulmonale
- (d) a pulmonary embolus
- (e) pericarditis

(2) Weight loss is uncommon in following:
- (a) severe emphysema
- (b) sarcoidosis
- (c) pulmonary tuberculosis
- (d) asthma
- (e) silicosis

(3) Features of respiratory failure include:
- (a) $P_{CO_2} > 6.7$ kPa/l
- (b) raised intracranial pressure
- (c) flapping tremor
- (d) confusion
- (e) peripheral oedema

MULTIPLE CHOICE QUESTIONS

(4) The following drugs should not be prescribed to an asthmatic:
- (a) β-blockers
- (b) cimetidine
- (c) aspirin
- (d) ephedrine
- (e) carbocysteine

(5) Rib-fracture may occur in:
- (a) severe asthma
- (b) carcinomatosis
- (c) pneumothorax
- (d) aspergillosis
- (e) tuberculosis

(6) The following appropriate in management of chronic bronchitis (uncomplicated):
- (a) breathing exercises
- (b) change of occupation
- (c) antibiotics during winter
- (d) oxygen therapy
- (e) help to give up tobacco

(7) Excess purulent sputum may occur in:
- (a) emphysema
- (b) fibrocystic disease
- (c) foreign body inhalation
- (d) lung abscess
- (e) fibrosing alveolitis

(8) Squamous cell cancer of lung is characterized by:
- (a) fast growing
- (b) peripheral
- (c) radiosensitive
- (d) cavitating
- (e) cause hypocalcaemia

(9) Steroids very useful in:
- (a) longstanding emphysema
- (b) pulmonary aspergillosis
- (c) Caplan's syndrome
- (d) late onset asthma
- (e) bronchiectasis

RESPIRATORY DISEASES

(10) Extrinsic asthma:
   (a) common in adults
   (b) allergy tests positive
   (c) hyposensitization should be considered
   (d) prognosis fair to good
   (e) eosinophil count high.

(11) The following categories of patient at risk from lung cancer:
   (a) heavy smokers
   (b) exposure to asbestos
   (c) exposure to carbon
   (d) positive family history
   (e) blood group B

(12) A child with chronic cough may have:
   (a) tuberculosis
   (b) cystic fibrosis
   (c) bronchial asthma
   (d) fibrosing alveolitis
   (e) eosinophilic lung

(13) Hilar lymph node enlargement occurs in:
   (a) bronchiectasis
   (b) polyarteritis nodosa
   (c) sarcoidosis
   (d) reticuloses
   (e) allergic alveolitis

(14) Haemoptyses occur *commonly* in:
   (a) chronic bronchitis
   (b) carcinoid syndrome
   (c) bronchiectasis
   (d) tuberculosis
   (e) sarcoidosis

(15) Elderly patients with recurrent lower lobe pneumonia:
   (a) may have achalasia/hiatus hernia
   (b) excess intake of paraffin
   (c) immunosuppressed
   (d) suggest reactivation of tuberculosis
   (e) due to fungal infection

MULTIPLE CHOICE QUESTIONS

(16) These are features of acute severe asthma (*status asthmaticus*):
- (a) bradycardia
- (b) hypoventilation
- (c) paradox
- (d) cyanosis
- (e) convulsions

(17) The following actions necessary if a chest X-ray shows an abnormal left hilum:
- (a) detailed history
- (b) lateral film
- (c) tomograms
- (d) tuberculin test
- (e) electrocardiograph

(18) Left diaphragm elevated on the chest X-ray:
- (a) may suggest pulmonary embolus
- (b) due to ascites
- (c) liver enlargement
- (d) large spleen
- (e) previous phrenic crush

(19) Nervous system very rarely involved in:
- (a) sarcoidosis
- (b) tuberculosis
- (c) bronchiectasis
- (d) hypercapnia
- (e) carcinoid syndrome

(20) 'Joints' may be affected in:
- (a) lung carcinoma
- (b) pneumonia
- (c) fibrosing alveolitis
- (d) asbestosis
- (e) secondary polycythaemia

RESPIRATORY DISEASES
MCQ (ANSWERS)

1. (a) ✓ (b) × (c) × (d) ✓ (e) ✓
2. (a) × (b) ✓ (c) × (d) ✓ (e) ×
3. (a) ✓ (b) ✓ (c) ✓ (d) ✓ (e) ×
4. (a) ✓ (b) × (c) ✓ (d) × (e) ✓
5. (a) ✓ (b) ✓ (c) × (d) × (e) ×
6. (a) ✓ (b) × (c) × (d) × (e) ✓
7. (a) × (b) ✓ (c) ✓ (d) ✓ (e) ×
8. (a) × (b) × (c) × (d) ✓ (e) ×
9. (a) × (b) ✓ (c) × (d) ✓ (e) ×
10. (a) × (b) ✓ (c) ✓ (d) ✓ (e) ✓
11. (a) ✓ (b) ✓ (c) × (d) ✓ (e) ×
12. (a) ✓ (b) ✓ (c) ✓ (d) × (e) ✓
13. (a) × (b) × (c) ✓ (d) ✓ (e) ×
14. (a) × (b) × (c) ✓ (d) ✓ (e) ×
15. (a) ✓ (b) ✓ (c) ✓ (d) × (e) ×
16. (a) × (b) × (c) ✓ (d) × (e) ×
17. (a) ✓ (b) ✓ (c) ✓ (d) × (e) ×
18. (a) ✓ (b) ✓ (c) × (d) ✓ (e) ✓
19. (a) ✓ (b) × (c) × (d) × (e) ✓
20. (a) ✓ (b) × (c) ✓ (d) ✓ (e) ×

Index

actinomycosis 193
acute infections 168–80
  mortality and risk patients 168
  organisms causing 169
  types 168
adrenocorticotropic hormone (ACTH) in small cell bronchial carcinoma 104
adverse drug reactions
  anti-cancer drugs 121, 122
  antitubercular drugs 159, 160
  haloperidol 139
  nausea and vomiting 138
air pollution 127
airways obstruction and bronchiectasis 187
alcoholics and pneumonia 169
allergen testing 85
allergic alveolitis (Farmer's lung) 5, 191
  case histories 39
  features and management 199
allergy in asthma 85
allergy tests 13, 85
alveolitis
  fibrosing 204, 205
    case history 38
    lung function 205
    management 205
  lung effects 201
analgesia
  entonox 142, 143
  subcutaneous infusions 143, 144
  terminal illness 133–7
antibiotics 66, 67
  antifungal 192–4
  pneumonia 171
  prophylactic 70
  terminal illness 137
anticonvulsants in terminal illness 137
antidepressants in terminal illness 136
antiemetics 138, 139
  continuous infusions 139
anxiolytics in terminal illness 135, 136
asbestosis 5, 38
  and mesothelioma 196, 198, 199
aspergillosis
  asthma 78, 192
  bronchopulmonary 192
    case history 39
  as complication 191
  management 193
  mycetoma 192
  organism source 191
asthma
  acute severe 93, 98
    features 93
    management 94
    risk patients 93
  in adults
    care protocol 97, 98
    clinical features 81, 82
    definition 81
    differential diagnosis 82
    epidemiology, sex and mortality 80
    management 81
    types and features 81
  aetiology and management 4
  airways pathology 78

allergens 85
in children
  care protocol 96, 97
  lung function tests 80
  management 80
  sex and progress 79
  types and features 79
cough 9, 12, 14
deaths 5, 73, 79, 80, 102
  acute 98
  constant 95
  risk patients 96
diagnosis failure 4, 95
drug therapy
  acute severe asthma 93
  antihistamines 91
  chronic severe asthma 93
  compliance 96
  inhalers 86–90 *see also* inhalers
  nebulizer 92
  oral 90–2
  parenteral 92
elderly, care protocol 98, 99
emotional factors 86
exercise-induced, features and
  treatment 76
extrinsic, features and treatment 74
features 2, 3, 75–7
GP and hospital management 83–92
intrinsic, features and treatment 75
  case history, late onset 36
occupational aspects 85, 86
  features and treatment 77
  agents 77
quiet chest 121
rare features 83
risk cases 83
self-recording PEFR 4, 80
wheeze, features 25, 26, 177
Asthma Clinics 84
asthmatic syndrome, drug-induced 200
attendance allowance for terminally ill 146

beclomethasone inhaler and asthma 89
Bencard Diagnostic Set 85
betamethasone inhaler in asthma 89
blue bloaters 64
Börnholm disease
  case history 34
  management 178
breathlessness (dyspnoea)
  acute nocturnal 28
  causes 26, 27
  constant, causes 27

control in terminally ill 139, 140
psychogenic, disproportionate 27
bronchial adenoma 39, 100
bronchial carcinoma
  adenocarcinoma, features and
    survival 105
  blood tests 113
  case history 36
  causal factors 101
  chemotherapy 119–23
    drugs used 120
    hair loss 121
    marrow toxicity 121
    mouth ulcers 122
    nausea 121
    side effects 121, 122
  cough 15, 124
  diagnostic features 107
  emergency 112
  hospital referral, indications 111, 112
  immunotherapy 123
  informing patients 125, 126
  investigations 111, 113
  large cell anaplastic, features and
    survival 106
  malignant pleural effusions 122, 123
  mortality
    and incidence 6
    sex 102, 127
  nervous and endocrine involvement 108
  palliative treatment 124
  radiology findings 109, 110
  radiotherapy 123
  second primary risk 119
  small cell, features and survival 104
    chemotherapy 120
  squamous cell, features and survival 103
  supportive therapy 124
  survival 101, 103–7, 114, 115
    factors affecting 117, 118
  symptom management
    cough 124
    haemoptysis 124
    pain 125
    psychological 125
  terminal care *see* terminal care
  TNM classification 114
  treatment, surgery 113–19
    lobectomy 115
    pneumonectomy 115, 116
    problems and complications 117, 118
    sleeve resection 116
    surgical mortality 115
    wedge resection 116
  unusual presentation 108
  wheeze features 26

bronchiectasis
  acquired, types 183
  airway assessment 187
  antibiotic prophylaxis 187, 188
  bronchogram 184, 185
  case history 34
  clinical features 184
  congenital 182
  cough 12, 14
  and cystic fibrosis 182, 183
  definition 181
  drug therapy 186
  features 2, 3, 182
  kidney involvement 184
  organisms involved 186
  physiotherapy 188
  sputum features 185
  surgery 185, 186
  wheeze features 25, 26
bronchitis, acute
  age effects 176
  and asthma 177
  management and drugs 176
  recurrent 177
bronchitis, chronic
  age of onset 2
  blue bloater 64
  case history 37, 38
  cough 10, 12, 14
  definition 59
  investigations 62, 63
  mortality 102
  pathology 61
  symptoms and signs 61
    predominant 64
  treatment 65–72
    bronchodilators 67, 68
    infections and antibiotics 66, 67
    mucolytic agents 71, 72
    oxygen use 69, 70
    physiotherapy 70
    problems 63, 64
    prophylaxis 70
    steroid use 68, 69
  wheeze features 26
bronchodilators 67, 68
bronchopleural fistula 118

Caplan's syndrome 195, 201
case histories, respiratory diseases 32–41
catarrh
  age and prevalence 53
  assessment 55
  children 53–8
  definition 53

  features and clinical types 54
  management and surgery 55
  treatment plan 54, 55
chemotherapy
  drugs used 120
  side effects 120–2
chest injuries
  management and treatment 209
  types 209
chest pain
  cardiac causes 29
  respiratory disorders 29
choriocarcinoma, case history of disseminated 41
chronic obstructive airways disorders
  causes 60
  features and types 2, 3, 59
  mortality and age 60
co-analgesics 135–7
coccidiomycosis 194
cold, management plan 56
collagen disorders 201–4
contact tracing in tuberculosis 157
cor pulmonare
  asthma 4
  case history 37
cough
  allergy tests 13
  bronchial carcinoma 15, 24
  complications 11
  crackles 13
  features in children 9, 15
  investigations 12
  management 15, 16
    scheme 56
  monophonic and polyphonic 12
  nervous 10, 15
  productive and non-productive 11
  smoking 10
  suppressants 16
  tests 13, 14
  types 14, 15
  viral cause 10, 15
croup
  features and management 57
  features and significance 18
  management 19
cryptococcosis 193
Cushing's disease 104, 108
cystic fibrosis of the pancreas
  complications 190
  features 189
  incidence 188
  inheritance 188
  management 189
  pathology and organisms 189

prognosis 191
sweat test 188
treatment and aims 190
dextrocardia 186
disseminated malignancy, case history 37, 38
drugs, lung effects 200, 201

electrocardiography, bronchitis and emphysema 63
emergencies 206–11
emphysema
  age of onset 2
  α_1-antitrypsin deficient 65
  case history 37
  cough 14
  definition 59
  family screening 65
  investigations 62, 63
  pathology 60
  pink puffer 64
  symptoms and signs 61
    predominant 64, 65
  treatment 65–72
    bronchodilator use 67, 68
    infections and antibiotics 66, 67
    oxygen use 69, 70
    problems 63, 64
    prophylaxis 70
    steroid use 68, 69
    surgery 70, 71
empyema thoracis 118
eosinophilic granuloma, asthma 78
epiglottitis 18
  treatment 19
erythema nodosum and sarcoidosis 163
ethambutol in tuberculosis 159

Farmer's lung 191 see also allergic alveolitis
fenoterol inhaler in asthma 88
flail chest 44
flow volume loops
  obstruction types 24, 25
  upper and lower respiratory disorders 24
foreign body 34
  cough 11, 12
fungal infections 191–4

glandular fever, sore throat 17, 18
gynaecomastia 46
  large cell anaplastic carcinoma 106

haemoptysis
  age and smoking 32
  bronchial carcinoma 112, 124
  causes and pain 29, 30

children and adult 31
  management 30
  specialist referral 31
  sputum tests 30
  X-ray 30
heart failure, cough 15
heart shadows, radiology 45, 47
histoplasmosis 194
hydrocortisone, parenteral in asthma 92
  acute severe asthma 94

immunoglobulin, IgE in asthma 74, 76
immunological deficiency, pneumonia mortality 172
immunological disorders 6, 7
influenza
  features 7
  and flu-like disease 19
  management 19, 20
  significance 19
inhalers in asthma
  β-agonist drugs and effectiveness 88
  anticholinergic drugs 89
  combination drugs 89
  sodium cromoglycate 90
  steroids 89
  types 87
isoniazid in tuberculosis 159

Kartagener's syndrome 182, 183
Kveim/Silzbach test in sarcoidosis 164

laryngeal tumour, case history 35
left ventricular failure, nocturnal dyspnoea 28
Legionnaire's disease, cause and features 174
lung abscess
  causes and organisms 179
  complications 180
  investigations 180
  management and drugs 180
lung function tests
  bronchial carcinoma 111
  bronchitis and emphysema 63
  cough 14
lung sepsis with cystic fibrosis 188–91 see also cystic fibrosis
lung, trumpet model 87
lymphangitis carcinomatosis 110

Macleod's syndrome 62
mediastinum, radiological abnormalities 51
mesothelioma 196
  and asbestos 198

INDEX

features and management   198
mobility allowance, terminal illness   146
moniliasis   193
morphine dose and pain in terminal illness   134
mucolytic agents
   assessment in bronchitis   71, 72
   oral   72

National Society for Cancer Relief   147
nausea, cause and control in terminally ill   138, 139
nerve blocks in malignant pain   144, 145
   indications   144
   local anaesthetic   145
   used   144, 145
non-steroidal anti-inflammatory drugs in terminal illness   135

occupational lung disorders   5, 77, 85, 86, 195–9
opiate use in terminally ill   133, 134, 139, 140
oral contraceptives, pulmonary infarction   31, 38, 39
oxygen
   bronchitis and emphysema   69, 70
   long-term use   69, 70

pain
   causes in malignancy   132
   diagnosis   132
   drug control   133–7
      aspirin   133
      co-analgesics   135–7
      opioids   133, 134
      paracetamol   133
   management, terminal illness   132–7
   nerve blocks   144, 145
   post-thoracotomy   117
Pancoat's tumour   112
   radical resection   116
paramalignant syndrome   112
peak expiratory flow rate, smoking wheeze   24
pension in terminal illness   145, 146
pericardia, radiological abnormalities   51
pericardial effusion, causes   45, 108
pericarditis, case history   40, 41
pink puffer   64
pleura
   effusions   108, 202
      drug-induced   201
   fluid accumulations   50
pleurisy types and management   178

pneumoconiosis   5, 31
   asbestos-induced   196
   beryllium-induced   196, 197
   fibrosis   195
   incidence   195
   management   197
   silica-induced   196
pneumonia *see also* Legionnaire's disease
   aetiology and organisms   169
   bacterial, organisms and features   173
   case history   33
   mortality   102, 172
   mycoplasma   175
   pneumococcal
      after-care   173
      complications and mortality   172
      diagnosis   170
      management and care   171
   viral
      chicken pox   175
      cytomegalovirus   175, 176
      diagnosis difficulty   174
pneumonitis, drugs inducing   200
pneumothorax
   spontaneous   40
   drainage   208
   emergency   206
   features   206, 207
   management, home and hospital   207
   tension, investigations   208
polyarteritis nodosa
   asthma   78
   lung involvement   203
   prognosis   204
postural drainage   188
Pott's disease   154
prevalence, respiratory diseases   1
preventable disorders   7, 8
pulmonary embolism
   nocturnal dyspnoea   28
   septic   178, 179
pulmonary infarction
   infected   178, 179
   and oral contraceptives   38, 39
pulmonary infiltrate, differential diagnosis   164
pulmonary oedema, drug-induced   201

radiology   42–52
   abdominal organs   52
   abnormalities   43–52
   bony lesions   44
   bronchial carcinoma   103–7, 109, 110
      findings   110
   bronchitis   62, 63

cavities and abscesses 49
coin lesion 50
collapse 48
consolidation 48
diaphragm abnormalities 52
emphysema 62, 63
heart shadows 45
hilar shadows 47
indications for 43
mediastinal abnormalities 51
normal X-ray 43
pericardial abnormalities 51
pleural abnormalities 51
pneumonia 170
sarcoidosis groups 162–4
shadowing, basal, apical 49
   widespread 49
significance 42
soft tissue shadows 46
tuberculosis 150–3
respiratory failure, acute
   assisted ventilation 211
   causes and diagnosis 210
   definition 210
rheumatoid arthritis, lung effects 201
rifampicin in tuberculosis 159
ronchi, causes 21

salbutamol
   inhaler in asthma 88
   oral in asthma 90
sarcoidosis 6, 7, 162–7
   case history and management 32, 33
   drug use 166
      steroids, indications and dose 166, 167
   extrapulmonary signs 166
   hilar lymphadenopathy 163
   pulmonary infiltrate 164
   radiological groups 162–4
   reticulocavitating disease 163
   significance 162
scleroderma, lung effects 202, 203
smoking
   bronchial carcinoma 100, 101, 103–7, 127
      survival 118
   chronic obstructive airways disease 60
   cough 10
   haemoptysis 31, 32
sodium cromoglycate inhaler in asthma 90
sore throat
   ages affected 16
   in catarrh 57
   causes 16
   cervical glands 17
   importance and treatment 17

cystic fibrosis 190
   management 18, 57
sputum
   asthma stigmata 82
   bronchial carcinoma 111
   bronchiectasis 185
   bronchitis and emphysema 63
   normal production 11
   tuberculosis 156
squamous cell carcinoma 32
steroids
   co-analgesia in terminal illness 136, 137
   oral and parenteral in bronchitis and emphysema 68, 69
   in sarcoidosis 166, 167
stridor
   causes 22
   features 21
   test and findings 22
survival rates, bronchial carcinoma 103–7
   favourable factors 118
   and staging 114, 115
symptoms and management 9–41
systemic lupus erythematosus, lung effects 202

terbutalene
   inhalation in asthma 88
   oral in asthma 90, 91
terminal care
   carers 128, 129
   family and specialist 129
   financial care 145–7
   home 129, 130
   hospice 130
   hospital and cottage hospital 130
   physical aids 142
   understanding diagnosis 125, 126
terminal illness
   breathlessness, causes and control 138, 139
   catastrophes, management 141, 142
   continuous subcutaneous infusions 143, 144
   definition 128
   diagnosis 131
   dry mouth 140
   nausea, causes and control 138, 139
   non-malignant causes 128
   pain
      diagnosis 132
      drug management 132–7
      entonox 142, 143
   patient fears 141
   sore mouth 141
theophylline 94

oral in asthma 91
tranquillizers in terminal illnesss 136
triamcinolone, parenteral in asthma 92
tuberculin test 111, 156
tuberculosis
  anonymous mycobacterium 150, 153, 155
  BCG 157
  conditions mimicking 155
  contact tracing 157
  cough 15
  decline, reasons 5, 6
  diagnosis 156
  drug therapy 158–61
    combinations 158
    corticosteroids 160
    duration 157
    hypersensitivity 161
  histology 156
  hospital treatment 156
  incidence and significance 148
  management 157
  microbiology 156
  miliary 152
  mortality 148
    risk patients 149
  organisms causing 149
  patients at risk 6, 149
  pleural 153
  pneumonic infiltration 152
  post-primary 151
  presentation, unusual 154
  primary 151
  radiology 150–3
  reactivated pulmonary 40
  risk 6
  scarring and adenocarcinoma 105
  types, clinical 150
  wheeze 26
tumours, fungating necrotic 142, 143
tumours of the lung 100–27 *see also* bronchial carcinoma
  types 100

upper respiratory infections, age and management 20

ventilation, assisted 211
vomiting, causes and control in terminal illness 138, 139

Wegener's granulomatosis, lung involvement 204
weight loss, causes, UK 149
wheezing 3
  age and causes 3, 177
  features and management 57
  inspiratory and expiratory 21
  monophonic 21
    and disorders 25, 26
    tests and findings 23
  polyphonic 21
    tests and findings 23
Wright's peak flow meter, mini- in asthma 4

X-ray *see* radiology